THE BIG BOOK OF BABY-LED WEANING

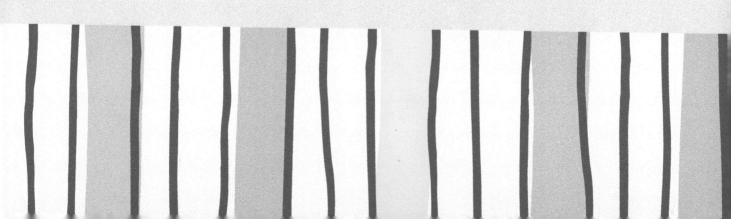

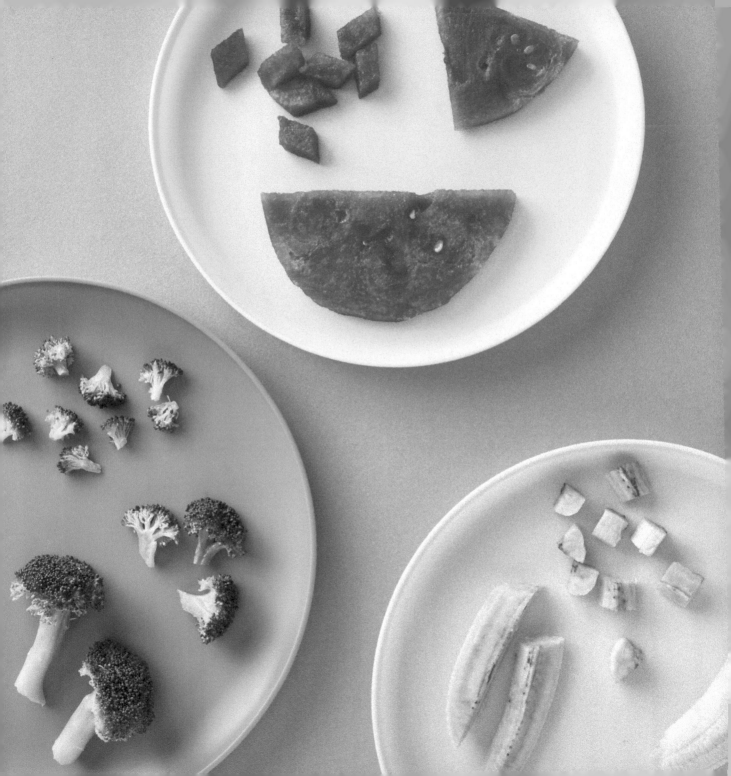

The Big Book of Baby-Led Weaning

105 ORGANIC, HEALTHY RECIPES TO INTRODUCE YOUR BABY TO SOLID FOODS

By Aubrey Phelps, MS, RDN, CLC

Photography by Laura Flippen

ROCKRIDGE
PRESS

To my beautiful children.

Learning to feed and nourish your growing bodies and minds has been,
and continues to be, one of the greatest honors of my life.

For general information on our other products and services or to obtain technical support, please contact our Customer Care Department within the United States at (866) 744-2665, or outside the United States at (510) 253-0500.

Rockridge Press publishes its books in a variety of electronic and print formats. Some content that appears in print may not be available in electronic books, and vice versa.

TRADEMARKS: Rockridge Press and the Rockridge Press logo are trademarks or registered trademarks of Callisto Media Inc. and/or its affiliates, in the United States and other countries, and may not be used without written permission. All other trademarks are the property of their respective owners. Rockridge Press is not associated with any product or vendor mentioned in this book.

Interior and Cover Designer: Lisa Forde
Art Producer: Sara Feinstein
Editor: Rachelle Cihonski
Production Editor: Mia Moran
Production Manager: Riley Hoffman

Photography © 2021 Laura Flippen. Food styling by Laura Flippen. Illustration used under license from Shutterstock.com. Author photo courtesy of Sarah Beirne.
Cover image: Blueberry Dutch Baby, page 95.

Paperback ISBN: 978-1-64876-423-3
eBook ISBN: 978-1-64876-424-0
R0

Contents

Introduction

Welcome! I'm so excited to have you here. I'm Aubrey, a Registered Functional Nutritionist, Certified Lactation Counselor, and momma to three earth-side babies and three angels. If you're here, it's likely because you're getting ready to start solids and may be feeling a little daunted. My goal is to make it less complicated and more enjoyable, and to support you as you help your little one cultivate a lifelong healthy relationship with food. In my private practice, I work with all sorts of mommas to nourish their pregnancies: caregivers to support the children under their care, and babies, to encourage their growth, development, and joy in eating. But, to be honest, nothing has prepared me better than learning to feed my own children.

Because I'm a pediatric dietitian, you might assume that feeding my own kids is a breeze. The truth is, kids rarely follow our carefully laid plans. With my first, I was *sure* that he would only eat finger foods, that he would feed himself, that I would never offer him a puree, and that he would be a champion eater. I was right about one of those four things. Although I offered a myriad of lovely foods, all carefully selected to meet his nutritional needs and expose him to a variety of textures and flavors, none of that mattered to my son, who decided he simply *would not* touch the food and feed himself. He had no issue with jamming any number of nonfood items into his cute 6-month-old mouth, but actual food? Nope. And oh, he was *interested* in the food, he just wanted *me* to feed it to him. So purees and mashes it was, until he turned 9 months and promptly decided spoon-feeding was *so* out and only self-feeding the most adult of foods was acceptable.

Then my oldest daughter arrived. She was born premature, struggled to simply suck and swallow while remembering to breathe, never nursed, barely took a bottle, and required a feeding tube for the first 19 months of her life. When we finally started solids orally, she wanted absolutely *nothing* to do with anyone feeding her other than herself. And so we had an entirely different experience with her than our son.

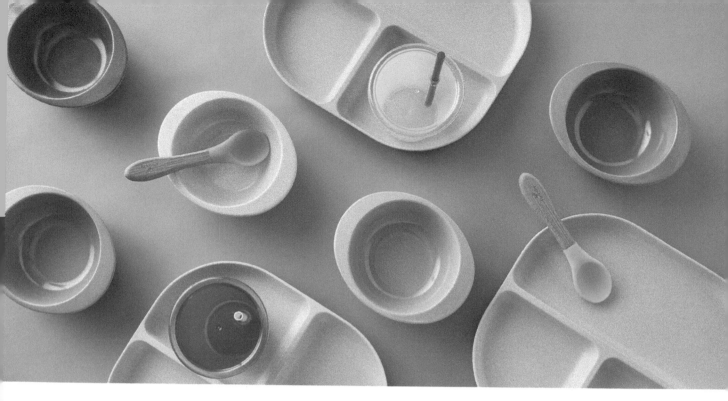

And our third? Well, she's an eating machine. She is the child who did what I imagined when I was still very new to the nutrition game and not yet a mother myself. But she threw us her own curveball, deciding to wean herself from nursing without even consulting me first!

My point? No matter how much you prepare, how much you think you know, or how well-intentioned you are, chances are the actual experience won't look all that much like you envisioned it . . . and that's absolutely okay. The goal of this book is to provide you with a framework for feeding your growing child. I'll offer some specific guidance and ideas, exceptions for bumps in the road, and more than 100 organic recipes. The recipes allow your baby to explore a wide variety of foods and flourish in their eating journey. Whether a food or recipe is an absolute hit or not, be patient, keep trying, and know that you are setting the stage for a healthy relationship with food, one of the greatest gifts you can give a child.

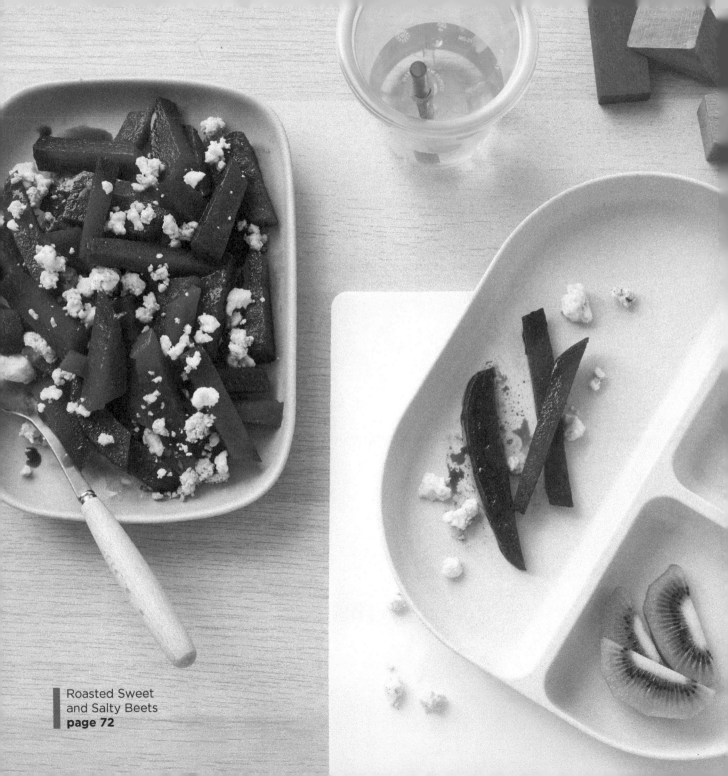

Roasted Sweet
and Salty Beets
page 72

CHAPTER 1

A Baby-Led Weaning Primer

Let's jump in! This first chapter is meant to help orient you to my approach to baby-led weaning, from the what and why to the how. Whether you're totally new to baby feeding or just looking for a refresher, this chapter will leave you feeling prepared and ready to tackle feeding your little one with confidence and excitement.

What Is Baby-Led Weaning?

Weaning is the process of baby replacing breast milk or formula calories with calories from food. The typical approach relies mostly on purees being spoon-fed to baby by a caregiver. Baby-led weaning (BLW), in its most basic form, focuses on including baby in family meals from the onset and emphasizes the infant *leading* the process.

The term "baby-led weaning" was coined in 2005 when it grew in popularity in the United Kingdom and New Zealand. This original approach focuses on baby doing everything. Only family foods are offered, in pieces baby can grasp and pick up to munch on independently. In this book—and in my practice—I don't use the term "baby-led weaning" in that strict, unyielding sense. My approach to BLW could just as easily be called "responsive weaning," where the focus is on allowing the child to lead by letting them self-feed, if and when desired, but also acknowledges that spoon-feeding can absolutely be "baby-led." (See "Blending in Purees," page 6.)

The Benefits of BLW

Why baby-led weaning? In this section, you'll learn some of the advantages, emphasized by a number of studies, of using a baby-led approach when starting solids.

Easy: BLW focuses on offering baby food from the family meal. No extra mess, fuss, or short-order cooking necessary.

Exposure to Diverse Flavors and Textures: Strict puree feeding results in a fairly consistent texture experience and generally pretty bland flavors, especially with commercial purees. A great benefit of BLW is early and frequent exposure to a variety of flavors and textures.

Self-Regulation: Children who learn to honor their own hunger and satiety cues instead of relying on external indicators of being "done," such as a clean plate or eating whatever their caregiver tells them they must finish, are far better at maintaining healthy boundaries as they get older.

Palate: Children who wean with BLW tend to enjoy a wider range of foods. When you offer what you are eating instead of catering to the perceived preferences of your child, they are more likely to try new foods and get the needed extra exposures to foods that take a little longer to get used to.

Motor and Oral Skills: Skills develop with practice, and BLW relies on the child to do a lot of the work, from grasping the food to coordinating moving it to their mouth and chewing. Because of the active role the child plays in mealtimes, they get more opportunities to practice multiple areas of development.

Eating with the Family: BLW emphasizes family meals. There are countless studies showing family meals support everything from better eating habits and less picky eating to less anxious and more engaged kids. I will discuss portioning for baby later in the chapter (see page 6).

FOOD = FUN

Starting solids can feel like a lot of pressure. You want to make sure you do it "right." There are a few nutrients you will want to make sure to give baby in order to meet their needs, but by and large the early stages of weaning are about exploration, exposure, and fun. And especially with BLW, that fun can be pretty messy. Try to focus less on what actually gets eaten and more on the experience itself. Eating isn't for nourishing just the body, but also the soul. Enjoy watching your little one explore new foods and smile with delight at the feel of an avocado mashed between their little fingers or the explosion of color when they paint that bright tomato sauce across their tray. Calm, unpressured, respectful family meals provide a strong foundation for lifelong happy, healthy eaters.

Let's Eat!

Your pediatrician uttered those magic words, "You can start solids." Congratulations! It might seem overwhelming, but rest assured that feeding your baby doesn't have to be complicated or difficult. Whether this is your first baby or your fourth, getting your little one off to a healthy, happy start with food and nutrition is probably easier than you think. My goal is to make this process as painless, fun, and simple as possible.

Ages and Stages

In general, the recommendation is to wait until your baby is about 6 months old to begin introducing solids (or six months from their due date, if baby was born prematurely). From a physiological standpoint, there are multiple reasons to wait until that 6-month mark.

First, at around 6 months, a breastfed baby's need for iron and zinc starts to outpace what breast milk provides, suggesting that the introduction of solids rich in these minerals makes physiological sense. For formula-fed babies, these nutrients aren't as much of a concern, because formula is designed to meet baby's needs. But research suggests babies are more receptive to new flavors and textures in the 6-to-10-month age range and that exposure to allergens during this period may reduce the risk of sensitivities developing.

Second, babies are born with immature digestive tracts. Although some babies' digestive tracts may be sufficiently matured to eat solids by 4 months, the linings of nearly all children's digestive tracts are ready by 6 months. Similarly, your baby's digestive enzymes develop over time, improving their readiness for solids right around that 6-month mark.

Finally, this time is a prime opportunity to expose baby to a variety of textures and flavors with little pressure for actual consumption. Babies this age are generally receptive to new flavors, and if little is ingested, that's okay—their primary source of nutrition will continue to be breast milk or formula until they are nearly a year old.

Starting solids at about 6 months gives baby's body time to adjust to eating and also takes advantage of their innate curiosity and interest in exploring. It also allows for lots of practice before it's necessary for them to be eating a sizeable amount. In other words, practice makes perfect, and babies this age *love* to practice eating.

Signs of Readiness

Are your baby's eyes following your fork from your plate to your mouth with rapt attention? Are they mimicking your chewing as you enjoy your meal?

These are indicators your child is preparing to officially join you at the table, but there are some other important signs to look for to ensure that your child is ready for solid food. Before starting solids of any sort, your baby should be able to do four things:

1. Sit fairly independently

2. Have good head control

3. Show an inherent interest in food

4. Grab and bring offered foods to their mouth unassisted

A baby exhibiting these signs is more likely to be internally ready to handle solids, and it will also be safer to do so. (Exceptions may include babies with a medical condition that delays coordination or muscle control, causes low muscle tone, and so on.)

It's crucial to keep your child's age and other signs of readiness in mind. Being able to hold their torso and head up in a stable position is vital to ensuring your child stays safe when exploring solids and greatly reduces a choking risk (see page 13). Do not rely on your child reaching a certain weight, the quantity of formula or breast milk they consume, or begging for food as indicators of readiness. Check out more signs of readiness in "Meals and Milestones" (page 9).

BLENDING IN PUREES

BLW is not the be-all and end-all for offering solids. Respecting your child's cues, regardless of whether you're bottle-, breast-, or spoon-feeding, is *the* most important part of the eating relationship with your child. Furthermore, if your little one has multiple caregivers, you may find that some of the people involved in feeding your child may be unfamiliar with and intimidated by BLW.

Whether you decide to do a combination of finger foods and purees, or straight purees with an adult spoon-feeding them, your child can still become a happy, healthy eater as long as the caregiver involved is respecting their cues. Allowing baby to explore with good teething toys encourages chewing practice and can assist in reducing an oversensitive gag reflex. Offering a wide variety of flavors, even in purees, will help develop a more diverse palate, and blending or mashing up family foods can get baby acclimated to the flavors at the typical family table so they're more prepared when they (and you) are ready to move to more finger food options.

When spoon-feeding, I recommend smaller spoons (see Resources, page 196). A spoon with a flatter bowl can also make it easier for baby to get the puree off the spoon. Be sure to offer small amounts at a time so baby doesn't get overwhelmed with a huge mouthful; think about placing the spoon at the front of the mouth, with slight downward pressure on the tongue, to encourage baby to wrap their lips around it.

Portions and Nutrition

At this stage, the most important thing you can do to cultivate a happy, healthy eater is to have fun with the eating process. Some kids take off, inhaling food as though they've been eating solids all their lives; others are a bit more hesitant and may only touch, lick, or throw the food. These are normal behaviors for new eaters.

This is a time for massive exploration and may or may not immediately translate into actual intake. Follow your baby's lead. At these early stages, a teaspoon of food (about the size of the tip of your thumb) is a pretty substantial portion for your new eater. Babies are amazing at self-regulation. Your job is to offer foods that are nutritious and to follow their cues for when they want to be done.

BLW lends itself particularly to your baby's inherent self-regulation, allowing them to explore and eat as desired, without any coaxing or coercing, because their main source of nutrition will continue to be breast milk or formula. This is the time to enjoy happy, relaxed family meals and to expose your little one to a wide variety of flavors, foods, and textures.

Picky Eaters

One of the most common phrases I've found myself saying to clients is "the only thing consistent about little ones' eating is inconsistency." Nearly all children go through some phase (or phases) of selective eating.

With my clients, I don't call it "picky eating" until a child is over the age of three, and even then, I often don't label it as such. Why? Because it's normal behavior. To your little one, all foods are new foods. It takes many, many exposures to a food to form a true preference or dislike. Studies have shown that early, repeated exposure to a food drastically increases the odds a child will accept and even prefer that food. It can be tempting to say your child "doesn't like" a certain food if they've refused to try it or made a face of disgust, but I encourage you to change your thinking: instead of "doesn't like," say "is still learning to like."

Sharing Signals

It's tempting to try to get your baby to eat. It's exciting to see your child trying new things, and you probably feel pressure to "get it right" and ensure they're eating the "right" things.

Here's the thing: you can't make a baby eat. Nothing turns a child off from eating faster than pressure to do so. Your job is to provide a relaxed, safe, unpressured environment for your child to explore food at their own pace. If your child is turning away from the plate, the bottle, or the spoon, that's a clear "no thanks!" Respect it! Honor it! Likewise, a child leaning into an offering, reaching for more, or opening wide is clearly saying, "Forge ahead!" You provide the *what* (food options), *where* (place to eat), and *when* (a predictable schedule). Your child decides which of the items offered to eat, or if they eat at all.

You can improve mealtime communication with your baby by introducing some simple sign language like "more" and "all done." With repetition, baby will soon pick up on these signs and eventually begin signing them back to you, which can help prevent table tantrums and thrown food.

Children learn to eat by eating; the best way to support that is to eat alongside them, share the same foods, and let them watch you eat. Be mindful of your own eating habits—slow down, chew thoroughly, don't overstuff your mouth, eat a variety of foods, try new things, and comment on what you like.

Eating Family Meals

From the first food offering, your child can and should be part of the family meals. Yes, some foods in the meal might not be appropriate for your child, like typical choking hazards (see page 13), but usually it's simple to adapt family meals for your new eater. Initially, you might overcook a portion of the meal to make it softer for baby. For example, if you're having pasta, continue to boil a small portion longer than al dente for baby.

Deconstructed versions of meals are another great option. If you're serving tacos, the hard taco shell isn't appropriate for babies, and most kids are more willing to try foods if they aren't mixed together. So baby's plate might have beans, chopped tomatoes, a scoop of guacamole, a spoonful of ground beef, and shredded cheese. Later, your child can experiment with mixing the components together and eventually progress to trying the full taco.

MEALS AND MILESTONES

Babies develop rapidly over the first year. One of the features of this development I find most intriguing is the way in which their progressions seem to be interwoven. We see that gross motor skills such as rolling, sitting, and crawling correlate with shifts in fine motor skills, such as reaching, grasping, and pinching. In other words, chances are that as your baby starts to display proficiency in a new skill on one front, new skills on another aren't far behind.

Understanding the typical progressions of the first year in relation to your baby's eating and ability to self-feed can help give you a sense of when baby might be ready to progress to the next stage. Remember, these are averages: every baby develops on their own time line. Some begin language development before they make physical advances or vice versa. If you're at all concerned, always check with your pediatrician.

4 months: Many babies are rolling and have solid head and neck control. They may have developed the palmar grasp, or the ability to use their palm and pinky finger to scoop things up.

6 months: Most are beginning to sit unassisted or with the support of their own hand or hands. Their fine motor control is improving, and they're now using their thumb and palm to pick up objects. A more stable trunk and greater refinement in picking things up signals baby's impending readiness to join the family table. Large pieces and strips of food lend themselves well to baby's current skill set.

8 months: Almost all babies are sitting unsupported, and the classic pincer grasp, or the ability to use the thumb and index finger to pick things up, is starting to make an appearance (developing fully by 12 months). As baby's finger dexterity increases, utensils become a great option to further refine their skills. Additionally, baby can now pick up individual, smaller pieces of food that you avoided feeding them at earlier stages, as they outgrow the propensity to scoop up a handful of items and jam them all (dangerously) into their mouth.

Foods to Choose First

For many families, the food you first offer your child is something you will always remember. That can make it feel like quite the momentous occasion (and it is). I want to emphasize that, in general, the order in which you offer particular foods is less important to your little one's successful eating journey than the manner in which you offer it.

Top Picks

With all that said, there are some foods that I think make better first foods than others. Iron and zinc are two minerals that become self-limiting in breastfed babies. Meat and animal proteins like **egg yolks**, **liver**, and **smoked oysters** are naturally rich sources of both of these micronutrients and offer several other nutritional benefits. These foods also have superb textures for new eaters.

I also recommend getting started early with **vegetables**, as their bitter flavor tends to be less readily accepted by babies, and early consistent exposure is correlated with greater approval and intake in the future. In general, always try to choose foods that are as close to how you find them in nature as possible.

Foods to Avoid

Just as there are foods I recommend prioritizing in your little one's diet, there are some foods that both medical research and I, personally and professionally, recommend avoiding.

Honey: Due to the risk of foodborne illness from the *Clostridium botulinum* spores that are sometimes found in honey, it should not be offered to children under one year of age. After one year, however, children have developed the bacteria necessary in their digestive tracts to protect against these spores.

Cow's Milk: Avoid only the fluid kind. In other words, yogurt, cheese, and even a splash of milk in mac and cheese are absolutely fine. The concern here is baby "replacing" their breast milk or formula intake with cow's milk, which isn't nearly as nutritious. Additionally, cow's milk can interfere with iron absorption, increasing baby's chance of insufficient iron.

Choking Hazards: Discussed more on page 13, foods that are hard for baby to chew (often round) should be avoided; in fact, instances where babies have choked with BLW have almost exclusively been related to inappropriate, unsafe foods being offered. Top choking hazards include hard candies; dried fruits; round pieces or chunks of meat (such as hot dogs and sausage); raw fruits and vegetables such as apple, carrots, and celery; chips; popcorn; and uncut grapes and cherry tomatoes.

Sugar: No one needs added sugar, especially babies. In this book, recipes that need a bit of sweetness include maple syrup, dates, or another whole fruit source that offers fiber and additional nutrients. Sugar, corn syrup, and the like should be avoided.

A NOTE ON SALT: There's really no reason babies can't enjoy a pinch of salt on their food. Studies suggest just a pinch of salt can actually increase acceptance and interest in bitter foods like vegetables (and we definitely want baby eating lots of those). Although I do recommend avoiding sodium-laden processed foods, if you're making food at home and seasoning to taste, there's really no cause for concern. However, if you prefer not to use salt, you can certainly consider it optional in the recipes to come.

Introducing Allergens

Studies suggest breastfeeding exclusively for 6 months to have a protective effect in regard to food allergies. Current evidence further suggests that introducing solids and allergens *prior* to 4 months, or *after* 11 months, increases the risk of food allergies.

Where does that leave us? In accordance with the current literature, I recommend introducing the top allergens—fish, shellfish, soy, wheat, egg, dairy, peanuts, and tree nuts (with rice and corn becoming more common)—sometime between 6 and 10 months of age. There's no clear evidence that one order is better than another, but I generally like to introduce dairy, wheat, and soy at the end of this range. This has more to do with wanting to avoid dairy interfering with good iron absorption early on and the potential difficulty of digesting grains than with a specific allergy concern.

When you start solids, I suggest starting with something that is *not* considered a top allergen. Once baby has had a couple of simple solids without issue, then just start working your way through the allergen list. Try mixing some peanut butter or nut butter in with a curry sauce or thinly layered on a piece of banana. Hard-Boiled Egg Yolk (see page 54) is a great way to introduce eggs. Fish and shellfish tend to be wonderful early food options with their naturally soft texture. Yogurt is an easy way to test dairy, and organic tofu is a perfect soy option. Introduce highly allergenic foods one at a time, preferably leaving a day or two between new ones to help clearly identify any issues that arise.

Three final things to remember:

1. If baby showed a sensitivity or allergy to a particular ingredient while nursing/on formula, work with your provider to determine when and how to introduce it into the diet.

2. If there is a peanut allergy or other severe food allergy in a sibling or parent, work with your provider to come up with a plan of how and when to introduce highly allergenic foods to baby.

3. You can be allergic to almost *any* food, so always watch for changes or reactions, even if the food you're offering isn't considered highly allergenic.

Choking and Gagging

Choking tends to be the top concern by caregivers and health-care providers when it comes to BLW. The good news? Research doesn't seem to support that concern. Although caregivers utilizing BLW did report higher incidence of choking, this is most likely (1) a product of caregivers not knowing how to distinguish between choking and gagging, and (2) from offering non-BLW-friendly foods (such as raw apple or carrot). And, despite these reports, caregivers also noted intervention *wasn't* necessary. The child cleared their airway all on their own.

Because BLW introduces more complex textures and asks baby to manage the size of the ingested food more independently, gagging (certainly) and choking may be increased with BLW, but the risk of an actual danger is quite low if the right foods are offered. Please note that as baby gets teeth, foods that were previously safe (such as thick strips of steak or a nice tender-cooked piece of broccoli) may no longer be so, as baby can now break off pieces of the food without having the ability to actually fully chew it. (Don't worry, I'll make notes in the recipes to alert you of these things.)

Know the Difference

The first step to safe BLW is knowing how to recognize choking versus gagging. Here's a popular phrase that makes it clear: "Loud and red, let them go ahead. Silent and blue, they need help from you."

Gagging is a *normal*, *healthy* response by baby to protect their airway. Babies tend to have a sensitive gag reflex to *protect them* from choking. This is a good thing. It can look pretty scary, but if baby is actively coughing, making noises, with a red face, they're gagging. They may spit up, cough up food, or even vomit, but that's okay—they're simply "overresponding" to the threat. Here's the big thing: you will want to help if baby is gagging, but don't! Your interference can actually lead to choking. Let baby try to work it out. You can sweep the offending food out of their mouth with your pinky *if* you can clearly see it at the *front* of their mouth, but *do not* reach for anything at the back of their mouth, because you might accidentally push it farther down their throat.

Choking, conversely, is quiet, with baby being unable to make sounds or cough, and their face or lips may start to turn blue. This is when you need to get involved, and I recommend *every* caregiver take an infant first aid course *before* you start solids with your baby. If your baby is choking, perform the appropriate first aid for two minutes, then call 911, then repeat choking and CPR steps until the ambulance arrives.

Prevention

The absolute best way to handle choking is to prevent it:

1. **Make sure baby is ready to start solids.** Review the signs of readiness (see page 5).

2. **Always supervise baby when eating.** Have baby eat in a secure seat, such as a high chair, preferably one where their knees are bent and their feet are flat on a firm surface.

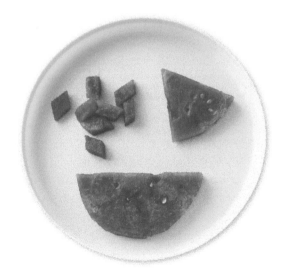

3. **Choose appropriate foods with appropriate preparation.** Pre-teeth, foods should be soft enough to mash with little effort between your thumb and index finger *or* so hard baby couldn't possibly break off a piece (such as a whole, large carrot). The latter is more for flavor, texture exposure, and gnawing practice than actual eating.

When teeth appear, those hard, munchable options will no longer be appropriate, because baby could break off little choking-hazard chunks. Cut foods into long, thin strips baby can easily pick up and control with their limited dexterity (about the size of your index finger, but a little thicker to start), moving to smaller, more bite-size pieces as baby's pincer grasp develops. Round foods, such as bananas and grapes, should always be cut lengthwise and quartered. Essentially, you want to make them as "un-round" as possible.

TRY, TRY AGAIN

The best way to encourage your child to eat a variety of foods is to offer a variety of foods—over and over and over again. Some kids love solids immediately. Others are a bit more standoffish. Neither is "right" or "wrong," and with rare exception, there's nothing abnormal about kids who need a little more time to warm up to solids.

If, however, your child is excessively disinterested or struggles with all textures by about 8 months, I do recommend checking in with your provider just to make sure there's nothing else going on. But, in general, the best thing you can do is keep meals calm, unpressured, and fun. Let your baby explore however much—or little—as they like. Remember, the vast majority of their nutrition is still coming from breast milk or formula, so there's no immediate rush to getting them calories from solids. And, pressuring them to do so is the fastest way to cultivating a "picky" eater and stressful mealtimes.

Keep offering different foods and textures, rotating through a variety of foods again and again so that no one food feels "new" or unfamiliar to your child. The more often they get to see, touch, and even try foods, the more likely they will start to enjoy them.

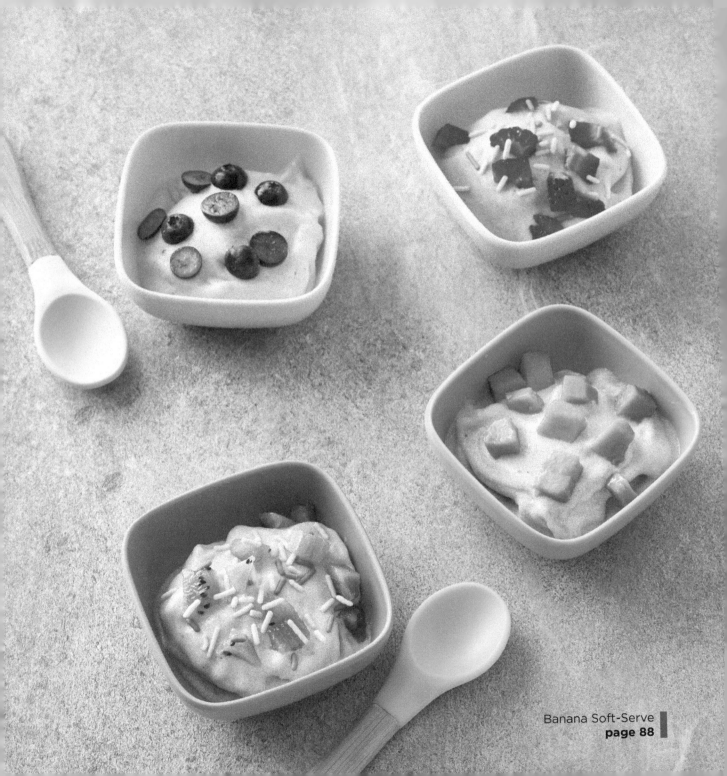

Banana Soft-Serve
page 88

CHAPTER 2

The Baby-Friendly Organic Kitchen

The best way to produce nutrient-dense, delicious meals for your family is to start with high-quality ingredients. In this chapter, we'll dive into the highest-quality ingredient options on the market, what to look for when grocery shopping, and how to balance wanting the best for your baby with not burning through their college savings. My goal is to give you the "ideal" kitchen scenario and at the same time recognize that it's just that—an ideal, not a requirement. Good nutrition is a spectrum, and it definitely doesn't need to be all or nothing.

What Is Organic?

By and large, organic is a great indicator of the quality of the item you're purchasing. In the most general sense, the "organic" label suggests products have been grown and prepared in a way that is as close to their natural, undisrupted-by-humans state as possible. For plants, this means no synthetic fertilizers, GMO seeds, or human-made pesticides. **In this book, assume nearly everything called for in the recipes (such as produce, grains, herbs, and so on) is organic.**

For animal products such as eggs, dairy, meat, and fish, it's a bit more complicated. Organic is good, *but* there can be superior "nonorganic" options (see "Certifications," below).

That said—I can't emphasize this enough—it is *always* better to get more vegetables, fruits, and whole and unprocessed foods into your child's diet than fewer, regardless of their organic, pasture-raised, grass-fed (or not) status. And good news: Organic is trending, with nearly all grocery stores offering a wide variety of organic options these days. Unfortunately, as we'll see briefly in the next section, earning the organic label isn't just time-intensive, it's expensive, too.

Certifications

There are several USDA certifications for organic, ranging from declaring a product "mostly" or "made with" organic ingredients to 100 percent organic. The requirements to earn such a label are rigorous, including keeping years of growing records, using organic seeds, avoiding nearly all synthetic pesticides or fertilizers, and having a clear plan for land sustainability, in addition to some hefty filing fees. For many small farmers, it makes more sense to invest in organic practices rather than the fees for the label itself. So, an organic label is great to look for, but getting to know the growers at your local farmers' market and asking them about their growing and feeding practices is a wonderful way to understand where your food is coming from and its quality.

Although "organic" in the animal realm suggests the animal lives in its "natural" environment, the reality is they simply have to have access to it. They can still be given feeds unnatural to the species, as long as the feed itself is organic. I recommend you look for the following labels when possible:

→ For eggs, pork, and poultry, **pasture-raised** is the gold standard; it means the animals didn't just have "access to" the outdoors, but lived as the animals naturally would.

→ For other meats and dairy (butter, yogurt, milk, and so on), look for the **American Grassfed Association** label, which means the animals had access to open pastures, were free to graze, were not given food with antibiotics or growth hormones, *and* were born and raised on family farms in the United States.

→ For seafood, wild-caught or sustainably farmed tend to be the best options.

Benefits

We're discovering daily how our farming practices and food choices radically impact our health and the planet's. Below are a few of the most well-researched benefits of eating organic.

Increased nutrients and antioxidants, improved fat profiles: Studies have shown organic and grass-fed/pastured products contain higher levels of many vitamins and minerals (such as A, D, and E) as well as more omega-3 fatty acids. Organically grown produce has greater antioxidants, such as vitamins A and E. Omega-3 fatty acids and antioxidants are key in improving bodily inflammation and growing a healthy, happy brain.

Decreased pesticide and heavy metal exposure: Organic foods reduce your exposure to chemicals, such as glyphosate and other pesticides, which are found in many conventionally grown and GMO crops, such as sugar, wheat, corn, and soy. These chemicals have been linked to some dangerous health issues, such as microbiome and potential DNA damage and endocrine disruption. Organic crops also contain lower levels of certain heavy metals, such as cadmium.

Better for the environment: Organic growing practices take into consideration the environment, focusing in part on sustainability, rejuvenating the soil, and rotating crops to help keep the land from being depleted. Organic growing practices also help save the bees. Bees are crucial pollinators: without them, the ability of crops to grow and thrive—and therefore the ability of humans to prosper—are under threat. Additionally, the runoff from pesticides, herbicides, and fertilizers damages aquatic ecosystems, encouraging algae blooms and disturbing the reproduction and health of marine life.

How to Shop

If you're not used to shopping organic, it can take a bit of practice to learn what to look for. Most stores have organic options for nearly everything these days, sometimes in their own special aisle or right next to their generic counterpart. If your store has a limited organic selection, you might consider ordering from some online retailers like Thrive Market, Misfits Market, and even Amazon.

Produce: Organic is often side by side with conventional. Some stores will use a different color price tag to identify organic options. If you're not sure, check the little sticker on the produce—those with a five-digit PLU (price look-up) starting with 9 are organic; if four digits, it's nonorganic.

Proteins and Canned or Packaged Foods: Meat, dairy, eggs, canned and other packaged goods will specify whether they're organic on the label, but check the ingredient list, too. Some companies don't get the official "certified organic" label, but the ingredients might all be organic. Remember when it comes to meats, dairy, eggs, and fish, organic is a great start, but certified grass-fed, pasture-raised, and sustainably harvested or wild-caught may be better. Look for BPA-free cans when choosing canned goods to avoid added toxins.

Label reading is a good practice to get into, as it helps you identify added sugars, hydrogenated oils, and other undesirable additives such as food dyes, high-fructose corn syrup, and artificial sweeteners. Try to fill your pantry and refrigerator mostly with items that don't even need an ingredient list because they're just what they are (apple, spinach, ground beef, salmon, etc.).

If you can avoid plastic containers, do, but I know this can be difficult. Just be sure not to warm up anything in a plastic container, as chemicals can leach into the food you're about to eat.

Spending and Saving

We've spent a lot of time talking about the importance of high-quality, organic ingredients, and you might be feeling overwhelmed about where to find all these things or how to possibly afford them.

This might be the ideal, but I'll be completely honest with you: We absolutely do not eat all organic in our house. We can't afford it. And just like at our house, it is far more important that you're feeding yourself and your children *whole, minimally processed* food than it all being organic. Choose the best-quality foods and ingredients that your family can reasonably afford and procure. The goal is to do your best, not perfection. And if buying those organic strawberries means you can't get any other fruit for the week, then it's far better to get more nonorganic fruit, just as it's vastly superior to get non-grass-fed ground beef for dinner than to get fast-food burgers.

The Clean Fifteen?

One of my favorite ways to try and get as much organic food in as possible while also being budget-conscious is the Environmental Working Group's (EWG) Dirty Dozen and Clean Fifteen lists. These lists are compiled after analyzing the USDA's Pesticide Data Program to determine which produce carries the highest pesticide loads. From this analysis, the EWG produces two lists: the Dirty Dozen, which focuses on the 12 kinds of produce with the highest levels of pesticide residue, and the Clean Fifteen, the fifteen least pesticide-laden options. The idea is that if you aren't able to go all organic, you could prioritize as many foods as possible on the Dirty Dozen list as your organic purchases, while you could forgo the organic option for foods on the Clean Fifteen list.

This does *not* mean that you should avoid foods on the Dirty Dozen list if you can't get them organically. It is exponentially, undeniably better to eat berries, even conventionally grown ones, than not, despite where they might fall on the pesticide list. So, if these lists are simply going to add stress or further complicate your shopping and meal planning, ignore them. Just get lots of fruits and vegetables, as many as you can. But, if you're looking for some guidance on when to splurge and go organic and when it's probably not necessary, these two lists can be a great cheat sheet.

And don't forget about frozen produce. You can often get a wide variety of less-expensive produce if you opt for frozen, which has all the same nutritional benefits of fresh. In some cases, frozen may offer more nutrients than the fresh because it was picked at peak ripeness and immediately preserved, but fresh is often harvested before its peak to make it last longer for transit to stores and sitting on shelves.

Canned foods are also a great option, especially for things such as fish and seafood, which tend to be pricey (just look for those BPA-free cans and no added salt or sugars).

Mini Meal Planning

Many families like a meal plan of some sort when baby joins them at the table. It can be especially helpful to prepare one for daycare or in-house caregivers. However, I want to remind you that one of the massive advantages and simplicities of BLW is that it really doesn't need to (and ideally shouldn't) require extra planning to include baby at the table.

The recipes in this book are designed to be a great option for the whole family, not just your newest eater. My best advice? Plan your own family meals and just focus on including something with the developmentally appropriate consistency to offer to baby (anything that can be easily mashed between your thumb and index finger). Eating is as much about joining the family at the table as it is about the specific food being offered.

Here are some simple ideas for foods to have on hand for baby, by age. Keeping some of these items available in the pantry and refrigerator make whipping up a baby-friendly offering a cinch. The lists build on one another; in other words, what was great at 6 months is great at 8 months and beyond, in addition to the other options listed.

→ **6 months (1 to 2 meals per day):** sweet potato (Rosemary Garlic Sweet Potato Fries, page 48), eggs, avocados (Simple Guacamole, page 41), banana, liver (Chicken Liver Pâté, page 52)

→ **8 months (2 to 3 meals per day):** broccoli, beans (Chickpea Mash, page 70), chia seeds (for "sprinkles" and Cake Batter Chia Seed Pudding, page 58), and ripe berries

→ **9 to 12 months (3 meals per day):** ground meat (Thai-Inspired Basil Beef, page 142, or Sloppy Joes with a Twist, page 114), cauliflower, cocoa powder (Double Chocolate Chip Veggie Muffins, page 90), canned green beans

→ **12+ months (3 meals and up to 3 snacks per day):** walnuts (Anytime Cookies, page 147, or Prune Bars, page 86), full-fat plain unsweetened yogurt, chickpea pasta, cheese (Sweet Potato Nachos, page 136)

Sample Schedules

On pages 25 and 26, you will find two sample menus for the week, demonstrating how to incorporate pantry staples and some of the recipes from this book. These represent how the schedule for two different babies *might* look.

There is no "wrong" or "right" here; although the recipes are listed by age, your baby's individual readiness, development, skill, and interest are all much more important considerations than whether a recipe is found in the chapter for 6- to 8-month-olds or 12 months and older. Some little ones have a lovely pincer grasp at 6 months; others won't have it until 9 months or older. Some children will be a pro at the straw immediately, but others might not be interested until a year or more. And if you're nursing, snacks might not be introduced until well past the one-year mark.

I included some puree options in one of the schedules, as a means to show you how BLW and purees can be so beautifully intertwined as you're juggling multiple caregivers and your little one's needs. The goal is to provide a meal plan that is nutritionally and developmentally suited for the age listed; however, more "advanced" food options may be perfectly appropriate for a younger baby—this is where your intuition and observation about your baby will come into play.

BABY A, 8 MONTHS

SUNDAY	Scrambled egg	Black Lentils with Squash and Herbs (page 76)
MONDAY	Avocado	Chickpea Mash (page 70)
TUESDAY	Cake Batter Chia Seed Pudding (page 58)	Ripe raspberries, halved
WEDNESDAY	Coconut Curried Kidney Beans (page 78)	Chicken Liver Pâté (page 52)
THURSDAY	Chia Seed Jam (page 68) on toast strips	Roasted Carrots with Pesto (page 49)
FRIDAY	Banana Bites (page 37)	Chive and Cheese Dutch Baby (page 79)
SATURDAY	Ripe pear, peeled	Classic Hummus (page 42) with hard munchables (large whole carrot or large piece of celery)

BABY B, 8 MONTHS

SUNDAY	Oatmeal with Chia Seed Jam (page 68)	Ripe pear, peeled	Chive and Cheese Dutch Baby (page 79)
MONDAY	Yogurt (add chia seed sprinkles)	Classic Hummus (page 42)	Grilled Salmon (page 55)
TUESDAY	Banana Bites (page 37)	Simple Guacamole (page 41)	Yogurt with diced ripe berries
WEDNESDAY	Daycare (puree)	Roasted Asparagus Spears (page 56)	Chicken Liver Pâté (page 52)
THURSDAY	Daycare (puree)	Rosemary Garlic Sweet Potato Fries (page 48)	Coconut Curried Kidney Beans (page 78)
FRIDAY	Daycare (puree)	Chickpea Mash (page 70)	Classic Hummus (page 42) with hard munchables (large whole carrot or large piece of celery)
SATURDAY	Hard-Boiled Egg Yolk (page 54)	Canned peaches (no sugar added)	Black Lentils with Squash and Herbs (page 76)

SOLIDS AND DIGESTION

Your baby is moving from a pure liquid diet to a myriad of new foods and textures. Some will take to it without so much as a blip; others may suddenly become fussy and gassy and need additional tummy support. All these scenarios are in the realm of normal.

Adding solid foods into the diet means that stools are going to get, well . . . more solid. Look for a still soft consistency, kind of like thick peanut butter or playdough. Formed is fine, but tiny, hard balls or baby straining and uncomfortable is a no-no. If constipation rears its head, focus on ensuring baby is getting ample fluids from breast milk or formula, offer water alongside solids if baby wants some sips, and try adding some of the "p" foods like peas, pears, prunes, and peaches. The recipes for Date Paste (page 40) and Prune Bars (page 86) are also awesome options. You want to continue to see four or more good wet diapers daily, and, ideally, a good stool every day, maybe every other.

Similarly, as the colors of the foods baby is eating change, so will their poop. Don't let colors of the stool throw you: red (hello, beets—these guys can cause pink urine as well), green (broccoli, asparagus, and spinach), or even blue (blueberries). However, streaks of black (unless they're kiwi or berry seeds) or mucus in the stool warrants attention and at least making a note. If it continues, worsens, or baby doesn't have a stool within three days after providing some prune support, it's time to check in with your pediatrician.

Kid Out Your Kitchen

Want to know the great news about BLW and the solid foods that are best for your little one? They are the same foods that you'll want to have stocked in the pantry and refrigerator for your own health, too. Remember, you're inviting baby to *join* you at family meals, not turning yourself into a short-order cook to cater to your newest table member.

Pantry Go-Tos

The list in this section contains items that show up in a lot of the recipes in this book, pack a huge nutrition punch, and are generally good to keep stocked in your kitchen. As often as your budget allows, choose organic produce and products, and grass-fed, pastured meat and dairy products, as applicable.

OILS, VINEGARS, DRIED HERBS, AND SPICES

- Olive, avocado, and coconut oils
- Balsamic and apple cider vinegars
- Sea salt
- Black pepper
- Ground cinnamon
- Ground cumin
- Ground ginger
- Onion and garlic powders

CANNED, BAGGED, AND BOXED GOODS

- Almond flour
- Canned coconut milk (full-fat)
- Canned salmon, smoked oysters, and sardines (oil- or water-packed are both fine)
- Canned or jarred tomatoes and tomato sauce
- Chia and hemp seeds
- Chickpea pasta
- Cocoa powder

- Collagen peptides powder

- Dried seaweed

- Gluten-free or all-purpose flour

- Ground flaxseed (move to refrigerator once opened)

- Lentils and beans (chickpeas, black beans, and kidney beans; dried or canned)

- Maple syrup (move to refrigerator once opened)

- Medjool dates (pitted)

- Nuts, creamy nut butters, seeds, and seed butters (no hydrogenated oils or added sugar; minimal salt)

- Oats (if you need gluten-free oats, check the packaging to ensure they are certified gluten-free)

- Salsa

Fresh Staples

Just like your pantry, your refrigerator (and freezer) should typically have some mainstays. This means that even at the end of the week, when you're in dire need of a grocery trip, you still have a couple of things available to whip into a nourishing, delicious meal. As with pantry staples, we aim to include as many organic fresh and frozen ingredients as possible. Remember to check out those Dirty Dozen and Clean Fifteen lists (See Resources, page 196) to help make decisions if all organic isn't an option.

ANIMAL PROTEINS AND DAIRY

- Beef, ground (ideally grass-fed)

- Bone broth, homemade (Slow Cooker Bone Broth, page 36) or store-bought (ideally from grass-fed, pasture-raised animals)

- Butter, unsalted (ideally from grass-fed cows)

- Cheese, such as string cheese, cheddar, mozzarella, goat cheese, or blue cheese

- Chicken, whole, and livers for Chicken Liver Pâté (page 52) (ideally pasture-raised)

- Eggs (ideally pasture-raised)

- Milk, full-fat (ideally from grass-fed cows)

- Yogurt, full-fat plain unsweetened (ideally from grass-fed cows)

PRODUCE

- Avocados

- Bananas

- Blueberries, fresh or frozen

- Broccoli, fresh or frozen

- Cauliflower or frozen cauliflower rice

- Fresh fruit (berries, melon, grapes, oranges, mango, etc.)

- Fresh vegetables (carrots, bell peppers, cucumbers, celery, etc.)

- Garlic

- Onions

- Spinach and other greens, fresh or frozen

- Sweet potatoes

Handy Tools

Just as planning meals for new eaters using BLW is fairly simple, so too are the gadgets necessary to make them. There are a number of great kitchen gadgets that can make prepping the recipes in this book a bit simpler. I've also listed a few baby-specific items that can be helpful, although they're not specifically necessary (see Resources, page 196, for brand recommendations).

- Bibs/high chair mats

- Cups (straw or open cups)

- Food processor and/or blender

- Glass storage containers (such as Pyrex or mason jars)

- Highchair

- Knives

- Measuring cups and spoons

- Muffin tins (mini or standard)

- Nonbreakable plates (BPA-free)

- Pots and pans (variety of sizes)

- Reusable silicone pouches

- Sheet pans

- Toddler utensils (BPA-free)

- Vegetable peeler

CUPS AND WATER

Starting solids is a great time to begin offering water. The idea is not that baby will be drinking any great quantity of water, but that you're making it a normal part of their mealtime experience and introducing them to a more "mature" drinking vessel.

Straw cups or open cups are ideal and better suited to cultivate proper oral motor function than sippy cups. Although your little one may enjoy some water during meals, make sure overall breast milk or formula intake isn't being impacted. Remember, solids and water at this stage are *in addition to*, not a replacement for, breast milk or formula. As long as your little one seems to still be getting their normal breast milk or formula volume, water on top of that is fine. This will change as baby grows and develops, with the expectation that when you start solids at 6 months, breast milk or formula intake really shouldn't change at all, but as you continue offering more solids during the day over the next 6 months, baby will slowly transition to nearly all solids by about a year. In general, I like to see babies up to a year drinking, on average, a minimum of 12 to 16 ounces of breast milk or formula daily.

About the Recipes

The recipes in this book are meant to provide you with tasty, nutrient-dense dishes for your growing baby, but are also appropriate for the entire family to enjoy. The chapters are arranged by age, with the simplest recipes first and the more complex full-family meals at the end.

Because I believe BLW is all about baby joining the family at the table, the servings listed for each recipe assume the whole family will be enjoying the dish or that it can be used in, or added to, meals for older eaters. If the recipe says it serves 4, that means a family of four, and 4+ means some leftovers are anticipated.

Remember, *you* decide which recipes are appropriate for your little one. Use the guidance outlined in the "Ages and Stages" (page 4) and "Signs of Readiness" (page 5) to help determine if your little one is ready for more complex offerings; but, more important, observe your child. Some kids will easily take to any of the foods in this book by a year of age, but others might still struggle with some of the later recipes by year two. Follow your child's lead and enjoy exploring new recipes, flavors, textures, and foods together.

The Banana Bites (page 37), Simple Guacamole (page 41), and Rosemary Garlic Sweet Potato Fries (page 48) are all great starter options. And don't be afraid to mix and match; try pairing a recipe from the chapter most appropriate for your new eater with other more advanced recipes in the book for the rest of the family. For example, the Roasted Broccoli (page 46), Rosemary Garlic Sweet Potato Fries (page 48), and Grilled Salmon (page 55) would be a fantastic meal for anyone at your table.

Let's take a quick look at some of the labels you'll see on the recipes in this book:

Dietary Labels: Every recipe includes a label to help you determine if it has any of the top allergens and if it fits your family's dietary preferences. I've included dairy-free, nut-free, gluten-free, vegetarian, and vegan labels and designated the following allergens: gluten, fish, shellfish, dairy, tree nuts, peanuts, soy, eggs, and sesame.

Tips: Many recipes include a tip at the end. These are meant to help guide you in making substitutions, figuring out what to pair the food with, or coming up with alternative serving ideas. If you see a recipe has allergens or other restrictions, be sure to check the "Tips" section of the recipe to see if alternatives are available that work for your baby.

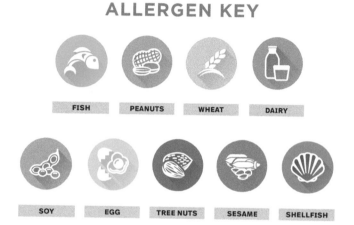

ALLERGEN KEY

FISH · PEANUTS · WHEAT · DAIRY

SOY · EGG · TREE NUTS · SESAME · SHELLFISH

Bless the Mess

Feeding babies is messy. Embrace it! Little ones explore the world with every one of their senses. Mushing that avocado around between their chubby fingers might seem like a waste or frustrating to you, but there's a whole lot of exploration and familiarization going on for baby.

You can absolutely remind baby that food stays on the table, doesn't go in the hair, and shouldn't be fed to the dog. But even with a clear boundary around mealtime expectations, there will still be messes. Bibs can help, as can eating in just a diaper when the temperature permits. You can even put down a high chair mat to help mitigate the mess and aid cleanup. Perhaps to start, make bath time a post-meal activity.

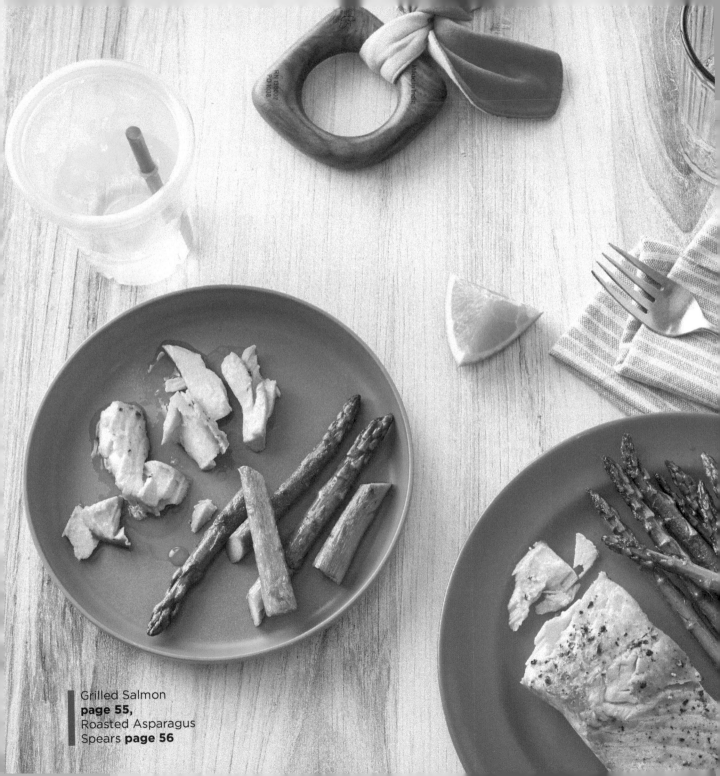

Grilled Salmon
page 55,
Roasted Asparagus
Spears **page 56**

Starter Foods (6 Months)

Slow Cooker Bone Broth

DAIRY-FREE, GLUTEN-FREE, NUT-FREE

MAKES: 8 to 10 cups | **PREP TIME:** 10 minutes | **COOK TIME:** 12 to 24 hours

Full of glycine and collagen, which are necessary for growth and digestive tract lining health, bone broth can elevate any soup. It's perfect for increasing nutrition in pasta, rice, or lentils instead of water and is a savory sort of "tea." Bone broth is best when cooked low and slow, ideally for 24 hours.

1 large sweet onion, unpeeled, coarsely chopped

2+ cups assorted vegetables or scraps (carrots, garlic, leeks, celery)

1 to 3 pounds bones (chicken carcass, beef marrow bones, fish bones)

1 teaspoon apple cider vinegar

1 (2- to 3-inch) piece fresh ginger, unpeeled, coarsely chopped (optional)

1. Place all the ingredients into a slow cooker. Fill the slow cooker with water, leaving 1 inch of space at the top. Cover, set to high, and cook for about 3 hours, or until the liquid starts to bubble. Turn down the heat to low.

2. Cook on low for at least 12 (preferably 24) hours. Turn off the slow cooker, remove the lid, and allow the broth to cool slightly, then strain the broth into 2- to 3-cup containers (glass mason jars or Pyrex work well; try to avoid plastic).

3. Allow the broth to cool completely on the counter before sealing with a lid.

4. Offer the broth to baby in an open cup or sips from a spoon. Store in the refrigerator for up to 7 days or in the freezer for up to 6 months.

TIP: For mason jars, leave 2 to 3 inches unfilled to avoid breaking the glass as the broth expands while freezing.

Banana Bites

DAIRY-FREE, GLUTEN-FREE, NUT-FREE, VEGAN

MAKES: 1 banana | **PREP TIME:** 5 minutes

Bananas are an easy first food. Try adding a sprinkle of peanut butter powder, a squeeze of lemon juice, ground hemp seeds, chia seeds, or a thin layer of nut butter on these sticks to mix it up. Quarter the banana lengthwise through the center, creating little sticks of banana about the size of your index finger.

2 teaspoons ground flaxseed	**1 banana**
½ teaspoon ground cinnamon	

1. In a small, shallow bowl, combine the flaxseed and cinnamon.

2. Cut the banana into sticks the size of your index finger. Roll each stick in the flaxseed and cinnamon.

3. For very new eaters, serve baby one stick at a time to eat with their hands. Store leftovers in an airtight container for up to 4 days in the refrigerator or cut them into chunks and freeze (for smoothies) for up to 3 months.

TIP: As baby's pincer grasp develops, feel free to offer bite-size chunks instead of sticks. The ground flax or hemp seeds can help baby get a better grip on the banana and also provide fiber, protein, and healthy fats. Many kids aren't huge fans of cold bananas; allow leftovers to come to room temperature before serving.

Watermelon and Mint Salad

DAIRY-FREE, GLUTEN-FREE, NUT-FREE, VEGAN

SERVES: 4+ | **PREP TIME:** 15 minutes, plus 1 hour to chill (optional)

Watermelon is one of our favorite summer fruits. This recipe plays off its natural juiciness and sweetness, adding flavor complexity with herbs and citrus. Even though this recipe calls for a seedless watermelon, please be sure to inspect any pieces given to baby to ensure there are no seeds.

1 pound seedless watermelon, cubed (about 1½ cups)

Juice of 1 lime

2 tablespoons thinly sliced fresh mint

1. Put the watermelon into a large bowl.

2. Pour the lime juice over the top and add the sliced mint, then gently stir to combine. Chill, covered, for 1 hour to let the flavors meld, if desired.

3. Cut up one or two cubes of watermelon into pieces about the size of the tip of your pinky finger. Allow baby to try to scoop the pieces up with their hands or preload a fork with one small cube at a time and let them self-feed. Store leftovers in an airtight container in the refrigerator for up to 3 days.

TIP: Try reserving a few larger strips or even wedges of watermelon before cubing. Sprinkle them with the lime juice and mint and allow baby to pick up the entire wedge or large stick on their own to enjoy.

Stewed Cinnamon Ginger Apples

GLUTEN-FREE, NUT-FREE, VEGETARIAN

MAKES: About 1 cup | **PREP TIME:** 15 minutes | **COOK TIME:** 10 minutes

Ginger and apples were made for each other. This is a great stand-alone option, but it's also delicious on top of pancakes, oatmeal, or yogurt or with some Dairy-Free Whipped Cream (page 59; store-bought would work, too). You can also mash up the cooked apples for a lumpy applesauce.

2 tablespoons unsalted butter

2 large Granny Smith apples, peeled and diced into ¼-inch chunks (about 1½ cups)

½ teaspoon ground ginger

¼ teaspoon ground cinnamon

Splash vanilla extract

1 to 2 teaspoons maple syrup (optional)

Juice of ½ small lemon

1. In a medium saucepan, melt the butter over medium heat. Once it's melted, stir in the apples, ginger, cinnamon, and vanilla. Turn down the heat to low.

2. Add the maple syrup, if using, then cover and cook for 5 minutes. Stir the apples and check for tenderness. The apples should be fragrant and easily mashed when lightly pressed with a the spoon. If they are not tender enough, cook for a couple of minutes more. Remove the apples from the heat and stir in the lemon juice. Allow the apples to cool.

3. Serve baby 1 to 2 tablespoons of the apples on a plate or tray to eat by hand or preload a spoon and let them self-feed. Store leftovers in an airtight container in the refrigerator for up to 4 days.

Date Paste

DAIRY-FREE, GLUTEN-FREE, NUT-FREE, VEGAN

MAKES: About 1 cup | **PREP TIME:** 10 minutes, plus 2 hours to soak

Incorporate this baby-friendly sweetener into muffins (in place of sugar), smoothies, oatmeal, and yogurt. Unlike regular sugar, it offers fiber, vitamins, and minerals. And, if your little one is having constipation issues, it's great bowel support, served "plain" or mixed with prunes.

1 heaping cup Medjool dates, pitted and chopped (10 to 15 dates)

2 cups hot water

Splash vanilla extract (optional)

1. In a small bowl, soak the dates in hot water for 2 hours. Transfer the dates into a food processor and reserve the soaking liquid.

2. Process the dates until chopped. Drizzle in small amounts of the soaking liquid as needed. Stop and scrape down the sides with a spatula. Continue to process until the dates turn into a fluffy, smooth paste. (The final consistency should be smooth and thick, not watery or runny.) Add the vanilla, if using, and process until fully incorporated.

3. Serve baby up to 1 tablespoon on a plate or tray for exploring with their hands, or use it as a spread or an ingredient in other recipes. Store in an airtight container in the refrigerator for up to 4 days.

TIP: Date Paste is a great substitute for sugar in naturally dense, moist baked goods such as quick breads, brownies, and muffins. It is *not* so good for things that are expected to crisp a bit (such as cookies) or be light and fluffy (such as cakes).

Simple Guacamole

DAIRY-FREE, GLUTEN-FREE, NUT-FREE, VEGAN

SERVES: 4 | **PREP TIME:** 10 minutes

This easy guacamole makes a perfect side dish for the whole family. For super-new eaters, spoon out a bit of the mashed avocado before adding the remaining ingredients, mix in just some of the spices, or cut a wedge or two of avocado and sprinkle seasonings over them to offer baby.

2 ripe avocados, halved and pitted

½ small, ripe tomato, diced (optional)

¼ teaspoon sea salt

Pinch ground black pepper

½ teaspoon onion powder

¼ to ½ teaspoon ground cumin

Juice of 1 lime

Olive oil, for drizzling

1. Scoop the avocado flesh into a medium bowl. Using a fork, mash the avocado to your desired consistency.

2. Add the tomato, salt, pepper, onion powder, cumin, lime juice, and a drizzle of olive oil and mix gently until well combined.

3. Serve baby 1 to 2 tablespoons on a plate or tray to eat with their hands or pre-load a spoon and let them self-feed. Store leftovers in an airtight container in the refrigerator for up to 3 days. (Storing with the avocado pit can help slow browning.)

TIP: Acidic foods such as lime and tomato can leave a little redness around baby's mouth—this doesn't mean baby is allergic. If the redness is only where the food touched the skin around baby's mouth and disappears quickly after gently washing with warm water and soap, it's likely nothing to be concerned about.

Classic Hummus

DAIRY-FREE, GLUTEN-FREE, NUT-FREE, VEGAN

SERVES: 4+ | **PREP TIME:** 5 minutes

Hummus is a naturally thick puree, packed with protein, fiber, with a dose of iron, zinc, and calcium. This is one of my favorite side to have on hand for dipping, spreading on wraps, or adding to bowls, like the Greek-Inspired Lamb Cauliflower Rice Bowls (page 180). Babies without teeth can use it as a dip, too, but if offering with a raw carrot or celery, the goal is for baby to not get any of the actual veggie but simply to use it as a vehicle for the hummus. For older eaters with teeth, carrots and celery are no longer a safe option.

2 (15-ounce) cans no-salt-added chickpeas, drained and rinsed

¾ cup tahini

½ teaspoon ground cumin, plus more for seasoning

Juice of 1 large lemon, divided

1 scant tablespoon roasted garlic, store-bought or homemade

Sea salt

Olive oil, for drizzling

1. Put the chickpeas in a blender or food processor. Process until well chopped, scraping down the sides if needed, about 1 minute.

2. Add the tahini, cumin, half the lemon juice, and the garlic. Process until smooth, scraping down the sides periodically, and slowly adding water as needed to thin to your desired consistency.

3. Taste and add more lemon, salt, or cumin to your liking. Transfer the hummus into a serving bowl. Drizzle olive oil over the top.

4. Serve baby 1 to 2 tablespoons on a plate or tray to eat with their hands or preload a spoon and let them self-feed, or use it for dipping. Store leftovers in an airtight container in the refrigerator for up to 5 days.

TIP: For homemade roasted garlic, preheat the oven to 400°F. Peel and discard the outer layers of an entire garlic bulb, and cut ½ inch off the top. Place the garlic bulb on a piece of foil, drizzle it with 2 teaspoons of olive oil, wrap it fully in the foil, and bake for 30 to 40 minutes, until soft and fragrant.

Pea Puree

GLUTEN-FREE, NUT-FREE, VEGETARIAN

MAKES: About 1½ cups | **PREP TIME:** 5 minutes | **COOK TIME:** 10 minutes

This recipe was a happy accident. I had salmon ready for dinner and . . . nothing else. So I started randomly adding some ingredients together, expecting very little, and instead got this flavorful side dish that I've revisited many times since. Fresh peas will also work; just reduce the cook time to about 5 minutes.

2 cups frozen peas

1 tablespoon unsalted butter

½ teaspoon minced garlic

Pinch sea salt

Pinch ground black pepper

1 to 3 tablespoons whole milk, divided

¼ teaspoon ground nutmeg

¼ cup fresh mint leaves (optional)

1. In a medium saucepan over medium heat, combine the peas, butter, and garlic. Cook for 5 to 7 minutes, or until the butter is completely melted, the garlic is fragrant, and a few of the peas are starting to caramelize slightly with a bit of golden-brown color. Season with salt and pepper.

2. Remove the pan from the heat and pour the pea mixture into the bowl of a food processor or blender. Add 1 tablespoon milk, the nutmeg, and the mint, if using. Process until mostly smooth, adding more milk in a slow drizzle as needed to keep the mix moving and to reach a fairly smooth but still thick consistency. Taste and adjust the seasoning as desired.

3. Serve baby 1 to 2 tablespoons of the puree on a plate or tray to eat with their hands or preload a spoon and let them self-feed. Store leftovers in an airtight container in the refrigerator for up to 4 days.

Simple Pesto

DAIRY-FREE, GLUTEN-FREE, NUT-FREE, VEGAN
MAKES: About 1 cup | **PREP TIME:** 10 minutes

Pesto is a great—and versatile—way to get more vegetables and flavor into a meal. Swap out the arugula for any leafy greens, such as spinach, kale, or dandelion greens, or swap in other herbs, such as parsley, mint, basil, or cilantro. Skip the seeds or substitute sunflower seeds, walnuts, or almonds for the pumpkin seeds. Please note: This is one recipe in which I absolutely insist you add some salt. The greens will be way too bitter for baby otherwise.

4 cups packed arugula

1 cup fresh basil

⅓ cup pumpkin seeds

2 garlic cloves

Freshly squeezed lemon juice

¼ cup olive oil

Pinch sea salt

1. Put the arugula, basil, pumpkin seeds, garlic, and a squeeze of lemon juice in a food processor or blender. Pulse until finely minced.

2. With the food processor running, slowly drizzle in the olive oil. Stop and scrape down the sides with a spatula, add the salt, and process until fairly smooth, about 2 minutes.

3. Serve baby 1 tablespoon on a plate or tray to explore or add the pesto to another dish to increase flavor. Store leftovers in an airtight container in the refrigerator for up to 4 days or in the freezer for up to 6 months.

TIP: I like to portion leftovers into an ice cube tray, freeze solid, and then pop out the cubes to store in an airtight container in the freezer.

Roasted Broccoli

DAIRY-FREE, GLUTEN-FREE, NUT-FREE, VEGAN
SERVES: 4+ | **PREP TIME:** 15 minutes | **COOK TIME:** 30 minutes, plus 5 minutes to cool

Vegetables can be a hard sell to kids; they tend to be on the bitter side, and babies are naturally predisposed to prefer sweet and salty (the flavors of breast milk). Remember, the earlier and more often you expose your kids to more "challenging" flavors, the more likely they will be to learn to like them.

1 to 2 pounds fresh broccoli, with stems
  (3 to 6 heads of broccoli)
1 tablespoon avocado oil

Sea salt
Juice of ½ lemon

1. Preheat the oven to 425°F. Line a large baking sheet with parchment paper.

2. Trim the end of the broccoli stems and use a knife or peeler to peel off any rough exterior skin on the stem. Cut the broccoli into large florets (about 2 inches with a 1-inch stem), then cut the broccoli stalk into ¼-inch rounds.

3. Place the florets and the stalks on the prepared baking sheet and drizzle the oil over them. Using tongs, toss the broccoli in the oil until evenly coated and spread evenly across the pan. Season with salt and pour the lemon juice over them.

4. Roast for 15 minutes, then shake the pan to help the pieces cook evenly. Cook for 10 to 15 minutes more, or until the broccoli is just tender enough to be pierced with a fork.

5. Allow baby's portion to cool, then serve baby a floret that is too large for them to put entirely into their mouth. Baby should be able to pick up the floret but just gnaw on the broccoli itself. Store leftovers in an airtight container in the refrigerator for up to 4 days.

TIP: Most roasted vegetables are best when cooked to tender-crisp. If you overcook the broccoli and it becomes soft enough for baby to chomp pieces off, I recommend cutting it into much smaller florets so you control the size of the pieces baby can put into their mouth. The broccoli "coins" from the stalk are best reserved for the adults and older eaters.

Rosemary Garlic Sweet Potato Fries

DAIRY-FREE, GLUTEN-FREE, NUT-FREE, VEGAN
SERVES: 4+ | **PREP TIME:** 10 minutes | **COOK TIME:** 40 minutes

I know it's probably blasphemy, but I actually like sweet potato fries better than regular fries. They are a lovely option for new eaters, make great finger food, and are the perfect side to any number of mains. You can omit the rosemary and garlic if you'd like, but it's truly delicious. This is a great option for introducing dipping sauces, such as ketchup, aioli, or Simple Pesto (page 45).

2 large sweet potatoes, peeled and cut into 3-inch-long, ¼-inch-wide sticks

2 tablespoons avocado oil

¼ teaspoon sea salt

1 teaspoon dried rosemary, finely chopped

½ teaspoon garlic powder

1. Preheat the oven to 425°F. Line a large baking sheet, or two small ones, with parchment paper.

2. In a large bowl, mix together the sweet potato sticks, oil, salt, rosemary, and garlic powder. Place the sweet potatoes in a single layer on the prepared baking sheet. Make sure there is space between the fries to allow for even cooking.

3. Bake for 20 minutes, then flip the potatoes and bake for another 15 to 20 minutes, or until they are golden and tender.

4. Allow a couple of fries to cool, then serve baby one or two fries on their tray or plate to eat with their hands. Store leftovers in an airtight container in the refrigerator for up to 5 days.

Roasted Carrots with Pesto

DAIRY-FREE, GLUTEN-FREE, NUT-FREE, VEGAN

SERVES: 4+ | **PREP TIME:** 10 minutes | **COOK TIME:** 30 minutes

This is a simple, vibrant side dish, but you can also just prepare the carrots without the pesto or spices other than salt and pepper. We love it with the more complex texture and flavor. Cut the carrots lengthwise into quarters, then in half to create about 8 (3-inch) sticks per carrot.

2 pounds carrots (about 10 medium carrots), peeled and cut into 8 3-inch sticks

2 tablespoons avocado oil

½ teaspoon ground coriander

½ teaspoon ground cumin

½ teaspoon dried thyme

¼ teaspoon sea salt

Pinch ground black pepper

½ cup Simple Pesto (page 45) or store-bought pesto

1. Preheat the oven to 400°F. Line a large baking sheet with parchment paper.

2. In a large bowl, mix the carrots, oil, and seasonings. Place the carrots in a single layer on the prepared baking sheet.

3. Roast for 15 minutes. Mix the carrots around on the tray, then cook for 15 minutes more, or until the carrots are starting to brown and are easily pierced with a fork. (You want to be able to mash a carrot stick easily between your thumb and index finger.) Add dollops of pesto to the hot carrots on the tray.

4. Allow a couple of carrot sticks to cool for baby, then serve on a plate or tray for them to eat with their hands. Store leftovers in an airtight container in the refrigerator for up to 5 days.

TIP: For a full family meal, serve with dollops of plain yogurt or sour cream, pumpkin seeds, avocado slices, and some sprouts as kind of a sheet pan salad.

Savory Spiced Black Beans

DAIRY-FREE, GLUTEN-FREE, NUT-FREE, VEGAN
SERVES: 4+ | **PREP TIME:** 10 minutes | **COOK TIME:** 30 minutes

This is a great dinner option to expose your child to some bold flavors and textures. Omit the cayenne for less spice. For little ones, I find a thicker, chili-like texture to be easier to handle than a soupier one.

2 tablespoons avocado oil

1 medium sweet onion, finely diced

1-inch piece fresh ginger, peeled and minced

2 teaspoons minced garlic

1 heaping teaspoon ground coriander

½ heaping teaspoon ground cumin

¼ teaspoon ground turmeric

¼ teaspoon ground cinnamon

¼ teaspoon cardamom

Pinch ground nutmeg

Pinch cayenne (optional)

½ teaspoon sea salt

1 (15-ounce) can tomato puree

2 to 3 cups water, divided

2 (15-ounce) cans no-salt-added black beans, drained and rinsed

1. In a large saucepan, heat the oil over medium heat. Add the onion, cooking for about 5 minutes, or until it begins to brown. Add the ginger and garlic and cook, stirring, for another minute, or until fragrant.

2. Stir in the coriander, cumin, turmeric, cinnamon, cardamom, nutmeg, cayenne (if using), salt, and tomato puree. Bring to a simmer, stirring frequently to prevent sticking.

3. Add 2 cups of water and the black beans. Stir to combine.

4. Bring to a simmer again, then turn down the heat to low. Cover and cook for about 15 minutes. Check the consistency. (If you'd like it thicker, remove the lid and continue to cook for another 5 to 10 minutes until the desired consistency is reached. For a thinner consistency, add some of the remaining cup of water.)

5. Mash 1 to 2 tablespoons of the beans slightly with a fork and allow them to cool, then serve them to baby on a plate or tray to eat with their hands. Store leftovers in an airtight container in the refrigerator for up to 4 days.

TIP: Try making this with Slow Cooker Bone Broth (page 36) in place of the water.

Chicken Liver Pâté

GLUTEN-FREE, NUT-FREE

SERVES: 4+ | **PREP TIME:** 20 minutes, plus 4 to 6 hours to chill | **COOK TIME:** 10 minutes

Full of iron, zinc, choline, vitamin A, protein, and healthy brain-boosting fats, liver is a great option for new eaters, both from a nutritional perspective and a self-feeding one. A thick puree like pâté can be a great way to get your feet wet with self-feeding and solid foods without the fear of choking.

1 pound chicken livers

1 shallot or small yellow onion, coarsely chopped

1 garlic clove, chopped, or 1 heaping teaspoon minced garlic

¾ cup water

½ teaspoon dried thyme

¼ to ½ teaspoon sea salt

Pinch ground nutmeg

5 tablespoons unsalted butter or ghee

1. Trim the livers to remove any white connective tissue.

2. In a large saucepan over medium-high heat, combine the livers, shallot, garlic, and water and bring to a simmer. Cover and turn down the heat to low. Cook for 4 minutes, then turn off the heat. Let the mixture sit, covered, for another 5 minutes, or until the livers are cooked through and are very light brown or show just a hint of pink in the center.

3. Using a slotted spoon, scoop out the livers, garlic, and shallot and put them into a food processor or blender. Add the thyme, salt, and nutmeg. Process until they are very finely chopped.

4. Add the butter 1 tablespoon at a time. Continue processing, stopping to scrape down the sides with a spatula as needed, until everything is well processed. Taste and adjust the seasoning as desired.

5. Scoop the pâté into one large or two small ramekins or bowls. Cover with plastic wrap, pressing it tightly onto the top of the pâté to protect it from air, and refrigerate for 4 to 6 hours or overnight to allow it to firm up.

6. Remove the pâté from the refrigerator 20 to 30 minutes before serving, if possible, to allow it to warm up slightly.

7. Serve baby 1 tablespoon of pâté on a plate or tray to eat with their hands or preload a spoon and let them self-feed. Store leftovers in an airtight container the refrigerator for up to 1 week or portion leftovers into an ice cube tray and freeze. Pop the frozen pâté cubes out and store them in an airtight container or bag in the freezer for up to 3 months. Thaw cubes in the refrigerator overnight before serving.

TIP: Forgot to get this going early enough in the day to set in time for dinner? Skip the bowl; spread the pâté in a thin layer over a large plate and refrigerate until cool (about 30 minutes). Not a big pâté fan? Mix a few tablespoons into ground meat dishes like chili or meatballs.

Hard-Boiled Egg Yolk

DAIRY-FREE, GLUTEN-FREE, NUT-FREE, VEGETARIAN

MAKES: 4 eggs | **PREP TIME:** 5 minutes | **COOK TIME:** 20 minutes, plus 15 minutes to cool

Full of choline, protein, vitamin B$_{12}$, healthy fats, and more, eggs are *eggs-traordinary*. For new eaters, I'm a big fan of the egg yolk, as the egg white can have a trickier or more off-putting texture, and is sometimes less tolerated than the yolk. Eat the white of the egg yourself, save it for adding to the top of salads, or use it in tuna salad.

4 large eggs

1. Place the eggs in a medium saucepan. Cover the eggs with cold water by 1 inch.

2. Bring the pot of water to a boil over medium-high heat, cover, and turn off the heat. Leave the eggs in the hot water, covered, for 10 to 12 minutes, depending on the desired doneness.

3. Fill a large bowl with ice water. Use a slotted spoon to move the eggs to the ice bath and allow to cool for another 10 to 15 minutes.

4. Carefully peel off the eggshell. Cut an egg in half and give the two yolk halves to baby to eat with their hands. Store leftovers in an airtight container in the refrigerator for up to 7 days.

TIP: Make the yolk a vehicle for flavor. It can be served plain or with a pinch of sea salt, fresh dill, a hint of cumin, paprika, or even curry powder.

Grilled Salmon

DAIRY-FREE, GLUTEN-FREE, NUT-FREE

SERVES: 4 | **PREP TIME:** 5 minutes | **COOK TIME:** 15 minutes

Salmon is an amazing superfood and a great first fish for babies, full of protein and brain-boosting omega-3 fatty acids. You can also do this on the stove, but the grill adds some additional flavor and makes the cleanup easier.

2 tablespoons avocado oil, divided

1 pound salmon, skin on, cut into 4-ounce portions

Pinch sea salt

Pinch ground black pepper

Juice of 1 orange

1. Heat a grill to medium-high heat or heat a large skillet over medium-high heat. Brush the grill grates, if using, with 1 tablespoon of oil.

2. Rub the remaining 1 tablespoon of oil onto the flesh side of each salmon fillet until well coated. Season with salt and pepper.

3. Cook the salmon, skin-side down, for 5 to 7 minutes, or until the salmon begins to lighten in color and the fillets release easily. Flip the salmon over and cook for another 2 to 5 minutes, or until the internal temperature reaches 130°F for medium rare, or up to 145°F, and flakes easily with a fork. Let the salmon rest and cool on a plate, skin-side up, for 2 to 3 minutes before serving.

4. To serve baby, remove the skin and flake into 1-inch pieces about the thickness of baby's pinky finger. Drizzle a bit of orange juice over the top and serve baby 1 to 2 tablespoons of the flaked fish on a plate or tray to eat with their hands. Store leftovers in an airtight container in the refrigerator for up to 4 days.

Roasted Asparagus Spears

DAIRY-FREE, GLUTEN-FREE, NUT-FREE, VEGAN
SERVES: 4+ | **PREP TIME:** 2 minutes | **COOK TIME:** 5 minutes

Cooked just slightly, so that it's still quite firm, asparagus spears are a wonderful side dish. They're easy for baby to grasp on their own and gnaw on. Don't let them get too soft, as this can result in baby gnawing off a piece. The goal is for baby to be able to gum a piece without actually getting much more than the flavor and juice or a very small, very well-gnawed piece here and there.

1½ pounds asparagus (16 to 20 spears)
1 tablespoon avocado oil
Pinch sea salt

Pinch ground black pepper
Lemon juice

1. Heat the grill to high heat or a large skillet over high heat.

2. Cut off the tough bottom inch from each asparagus spear and discard. Then, in a large bowl, toss the spears gently with the oil, salt, and pepper. Place the spears on the grill or spread them out in the hot pan.

3. Cook for 3 to 5 minutes, rotating periodically to cook all sides evenly. The spears are done when they're bright green in color and just starting to be easily pierced with a fork. Squeeze a bit of lemon juice over the top.

4. Let one or two thicker spears cool. Serve baby one spear at a time, whole or cut in half, on a plate or tray to eat with their hands; the pieces should not be shorter than 4 inches long. Store leftovers in an airtight container in the refrigerator for up to 5 days.

Breast Milk Chia Seed Pudding

DAIRY-FREE, GLUTEN-FREE, NUT-FREE, VEGAN

MAKES: About 1 cup | **PREP TIME:** 10 minutes, plus 4 hours to chill

Sometimes little ones get so excited about solids they start to prematurely cut their breast milk or formula intake. I often have to help families figure out how to continue with breast milk or formula until the novelty of solids wears off a bit. For older kids, you can substitute a milk of your choice for the breast milk.

1 cup breast milk or formula (check for dairy-free or vegan if needed)

3 to 4 tablespoons chia seeds

2 to 3 tablespoons mashed banana, fruit puree of choice, or Date Paste (page 40) (optional)

¼ teaspoon vanilla extract

¼ teaspoon ground cinnamon

1. In a medium bowl, whisk together the breast milk, chia seeds, banana (if using), vanilla, and cinnamon. Whisk until smooth. Let the mixture sit for 10 minutes, then whisk again.

2. Refrigerate in an airtight container or for at least 4 hours or overnight. It should be the thickness of a thick pudding after chilled. If not, stir in more chia seeds and chill for another hour.

3. Stir well before serving. Serve baby 1 or 2 tablespoons on a plate or tray to eat with their hands or preload a spoon and let them self-feed. Store leftovers in an airtight container in the refrigerator for up to 3 days if the breast milk was fresh, or 24 hours if previously frozen.

TIP: If you make this a thinner consistency, like yogurt, it can be served via a large straw or reusable pouch. Cocoa powder (½ to 1 tablespoon) can be added for a chocolate option.

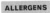

Cake Batter Chia Seed Pudding

GLUTEN-FREE

SERVES: 4+ | **PREP TIME:** 15 minutes, plus 4 hours to chill

Who doesn't want cake batter for breakfast? This is a tasty breakfast, snack, or anytime option. I like to keep a batch in the refrigerator to portion out whenever we want it throughout the week. I also love that it has omega-3s and spinach. For added protein and gut support, be sure to add the collagen powder. Try Ripple milk for a dairy-free option.

1 to 1½ cups milk of choice

2 large handfuls fresh spinach (about 3 ounces)

6 tablespoons chia seeds

¼ cup all-natural creamy almond butter

¼ cup gluten-free oats

6 Medjool dates, pitted and diced

1 teaspoon vanilla extract

¼ teaspoon almond extract (optional)

2 heaping tablespoons collagen powder (optional)

1. Put all the ingredients into a blender and blend until smooth. Stop periodically to scrape down the sides with a spatula, and drizzle in more milk if needed to keep the mix moving. It will be fairly thick.

2. Transfer the pudding into a large covered glass container and refrigerate for at least 4 hours or overnight.

3. Serve baby 1 to 2 tablespoons on their plate or tray to eat with their hands or preload a spoon and let them self-feed. Store leftovers in an airtight container in the refrigerator for up to 4 days.

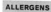

Dairy-Free Whipped Cream

DAIRY-FREE, GLUTEN-FREE, VEGAN

MAKES: Up to 2 cups | **PREP TIME:** 10 minutes

This is a quick and simple dairy-free whipped cream (and there's a dairy version in the tip) for a fun dipping option or just a delicious treat. We love it on hot cocoa, for dipping pancake and waffle strips, or as a simple "frosting" on muffins.

1 (15-ounce) can full-fat coconut milk, refrigerated overnight

½ tablespoon to 1 tablespoon maple syrup

¼ teaspoon vanilla extract

1. Scoop the thick cream from the top of the can of the coconut milk into the bowl of a stand mixer, leaving the coconut water behind. Add the maple syrup and vanilla and begin beating with the whisk attachment on medium-high speed.

2. Beat until light and fluffy, about 5 minutes, scraping down the sides as needed. Taste and adjust sweetness as desired, beating for just another moment until well combined.

3. Serve baby 1 to 2 tablespoons on a plate or tray to eat with their hands or preload a spoon and let them self-feed. Store leftovers in an airtight container in the refrigerator for up to 4 days. It will thicken up in the refrigerator; feel free to fluff it in the mixer again before serving.

TIP: For a dairy-based version, combine 2 teaspoons ground chia seeds with 2 teaspoons hot water in a small bowl and set aside. Substitute 1 cup heavy cream for the coconut cream and beat on high. When the cream begins to thicken, add the chia seed gel, then resume beating on high until stiff peaks form. Store in an airtight container in the refrigerator for up to 4 days.

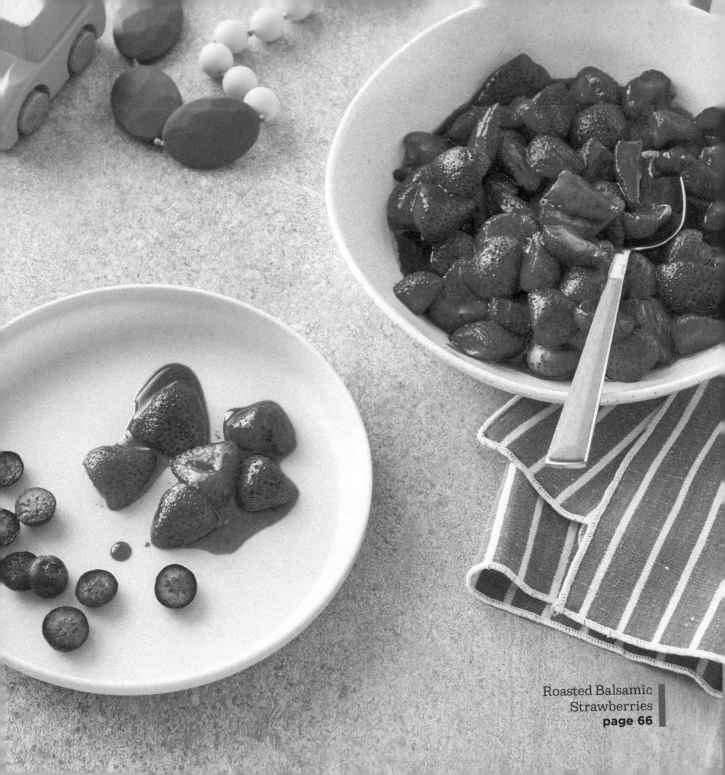

Roasted Balsamic
Strawberries
page 66

Level Up (6 to 8 Months)

Homemade Almond Milk

DAIRY-FREE, GLUTEN-FREE, VEGAN

MAKES: About 3 cups | **PREP TIME:** 10 minutes

Store-bought almond milks are certainly available, but I also wanted to provide some homemade alternatives. The only special equipment needed to make this almond milk is a cheesecloth or a nut milk bag. Remember, as always, when blending hot liquid in a blender, remove the small plastic cap in the center of the lid to allow steam to escape and cover the hole with a clean towel or paper towel to prevent a volcanic mess.

¼ cup raw almonds

2 teaspoons ground flaxseed

¼ teaspoon vanilla extract

Pinch sea salt

3 cups hot water, divided

1 to 3 teaspoons maple syrup or Date Paste (page 40) (optional)

1. Put the almonds, flaxseed, vanilla, and salt into a blender.

2. Pour about 1 cup of the hot water into the blender. Put the lid on the blender (remember to remove the plastic cap from the center and cover it with a clean towel or paper towel). Blend on low until well combined and starting to thicken, increasing the speed as you go.

3. Once thickened, return the speed to low and begin to slowly pour in the remaining 2 cups of hot water, blending until thoroughly mixed. Carefully taste the hot almond milk; if you'd like to sweeten it, add the syrup or Date Paste, a little at a time, and blend to combine.

4. Place the cheesecloth or nut milk bag into a large bowl and pour in the almond milk. Let it cool until you can comfortably handle the cheesecloth without burning your hands. Gently squeeze the almond mixture until you've gotten out as much of the milk as you can into the bowl.

5. Pour the strained almond milk into a mason jar or other airtight container.

6. Serve baby the almond milk in an open cup, or straw cup, or use it as a dairy milk replacement in recipes. Store leftovers in an airtight container in the refrigerator for up to 5 days.

TIP: The almond milk will separate in the refrigerator; shake gently before using. For a strawberry version, try blending in some Roasted Balsamic Strawberries (page 66) before straining, or add 1 to 2 tablespoons of cocoa powder and additional maple syrup for a chocolate version.

Homemade Oat Milk

DAIRY-FREE, GLUTEN-FREE, NUT-FREE, VEGAN
MAKES: About 3 cups | **PREP TIME:** 5 minutes, plus overnight to soak

For those in need of a dairy-free *and* nut-free milk, I've got you covered. This is incredibly simple to make and costs quite a bit less than store-bought versions. If you won't need the full batch, feel free to freeze leftovers or halve the recipe.

¾ cup gluten-free oats
6 cups water, divided
½ teaspoon vanilla extract

Pinch sea salt
2 to 4 teaspoons maple syrup or Date Paste (page 40)

1. In medium bowl, combine the oats with 3 cups of water. Allow the mixture to soak overnight on the counter, then rinse the oats and put them into a blender.

2. Add the remaining 3 cups of water, the vanilla, and the salt and blend until smooth. Taste and add the sweetener 1 teaspoon at a time until the milk reaches your desired sweetness.

3. Strain using a cheesecloth or a nut milk bag over a medium bowl, squeezing gently to remove all the oat milk but not push any of the sediment through. Pour the strained oat milk into a mason jar or other airtight container.

4. Serve baby the oat milk in an open cup or straw cup or use it as a dairy milk replacement in recipes. Store leftovers in an airtight container in the refrigerator for up to 5 days.

TIP: Check out the tip in Homemade Almond Milk (page 62) for variations on this base recipe. This is also delicious with a pinch of ground cinnamon.

Homemade Hot Cocoa

GLUTEN-FREE, NUT-FREE, VEGETARIAN

MAKES: 8 ounces | **PREP TIME:** 5 minutes | **COOK TIME:** 5 minutes

Hot chocolate is a fun treat or snack. We love making it for winter holiday walks or book-and-cuddle sessions. This is a great age to start introducing a straw or open cup, which is perfect for a slightly warm beverage such as cocoa.

8 ounces whole milk

2 to 3 teaspoons maple syrup, depending on desired sweetness

1 heaping tablespoon unsweetened cocoa powder

¼ teaspoon vanilla extract

Pinch sea salt

Pinch ground cinnamon

Pinch ground nutmeg

1. In a small saucepan over low to medium heat, warm the milk and maple syrup. After a minute or two, whisk in the cocoa powder, vanilla, salt, cinnamon, and nutmeg.

2. Keep whisking for about 2 minutes, or until the hot cocoa is smooth and your desired temperature. For little ones, I recommend checking with the tip of your pinky; if it feels warm, it's good. If it feels hot, let it cool for a bit.

3. Serve baby about 2 ounces in an open cup or straw cup. Store leftovers in an airtight container in the refrigerator for up to 4 days; whisk thoroughly before serving. Reheating is optional.

TIP: For a dairy-free option, use full-fat coconut milk or Ripple milk. If you've got pumped breast milk you'd like to use, feel free to substitute it for the milk.

Roasted Balsamic Strawberries

DAIRY-FREE, GLUTEN-FREE, NUT-FREE, VEGAN

MAKES: About 1 cup | **PREP TIME:** 5 minutes | **COOK TIME:** 35 minutes

Ripe summer strawberries are one of the best things about summer. Plus, they're full of fiber and antioxidants. I love taking my kids to a local pick-your-own farm every June. These strawberries can be eaten all on their own, used to top a special treat such as ice cream, or used at breakfast as a yogurt topper.

1 pound fresh ripe strawberries, tops removed

Avocado oil

1 tablespoon maple syrup

2 teaspoons balsamic vinegar

1. Preheat the oven to 350°F. Line an 8-by-8 baking dish with parchment paper.

2. Quarter large strawberries and halve small ones, then put them into the prepared dish. Drizzle avocado oil and the maple syrup over the top. Stir gently to combine.

3. Bake for 20 minutes, then remove the strawberries from the oven and stir in the vinegar. Place the dish back in the oven and bake for another 10 to 15 minutes, or until the berries are softened and their juices are starting to thicken and bubble.

4. Allow a 1- to 2-tablespoon portion to cool for baby, then serve it on a plate or tray for them to eat with their hands or preload a spoon and let them self-feed. Store leftovers in an airtight container in the refrigerator for up to 5 days.

TIP: For a special treat, try using these roasted berries in a simple smoothie. In a blender, combine 6 ounces of milk with ½ cup (or more) of roasted strawberries and ice, then blend until smooth.

Basil Nectarine Salad

GLUTEN-FREE, NUT-FREE, VEGETARIAN

SERVES: 4 | **PREP TIME:** 15 minutes

I love using fruit to introduce little ones to more complex flavors. Kids generally innately like sweet fruits, so it's great to pair them with things like herbs, as in the Watermelon and Mint Salad (page 38). And it's a great way to make a simple ingredient seem a bit fancier and more adult.

3 or 4 ripe nectarines, peeled and cut in ¼-inch strips

¼ cup loosely packed fresh basil leaves

2 tablespoons goat cheese, crumbled (optional)

Pinch ground black pepper

Olive oil

1. Put the nectarine slices into a medium bowl. Roll the basil leaves tightly and then cut them into thin slices. Sprinkle the cut basil over the nectarines.

2. Add the goat cheese (if using) and pepper and toss everything together gently. Drizzle olive oil over the top before serving.

3. Serve baby a few nectarine slices with the basil and goat cheese on a plate or tray to eat with their hands. Store leftovers in an airtight container in the refrigerator for up to 3 days.

TIP: Make sure you're choosing ripe, juicy nectarines. The flesh should yield easily if gently pressed. For older family members, this is delicious on top of a bed of lettuce with a drizzle of balsamic vinegar.

Chia Seed Jam

DAIRY-FREE, GLUTEN-FREE, NUT-FREE, VEGAN

MAKES: About 1 cup | **PREP TIME:** 5 minutes | **COOK TIME:** 10 minutes

PB&J is a classic. *But*, most store-bought (and homemade) jams are quite sugary, which isn't ideal. This is a super-simple and adaptable jam recipe you can whip up in 15 minutes. The chia seeds provide fiber, iron, calcium, and omega-3 fats.

2 cups finely chopped fruit of choice, fresh or frozen and thawed

2 to 4 tablespoons chia seeds, divided

1 to 2 tablespoons maple syrup, divided

Juice of ½ lemon

1. In a medium saucepan, heat the chopped fruit over medium heat for about 2 minutes, or until warmed through. Mash the fruit to your desired consistency.

2. Add 2 tablespoons of chia seeds, 1 tablespoon of syrup, and the lemon juice. Stir to combine and bring to a simmer. Cook for another 2 or 3 minutes, until the jam starts to thicken.

3. Remove the pan from the heat and let it sit for 5 minutes. Stir and check the consistency and sweetness. If you'd like to adjust either, add more chia seeds or maple syrup, 1 teaspoon at a time.

4. Make sure the jam has cooled, then serve baby 1 to 2 tablespoons on a plate or tray or preload a spoon and let them self-feed. Store leftovers in an airtight container in the refrigerator for up to 5 days.

TIP: Grapes, cherries, strawberries, raspberries, peeled peaches . . . try any of them. (I'd avoid using oranges, apple, pear, and banana for this recipe.) Swirl some jam into yogurt or oatmeal for flavor and sweetness, or make a classic PB&J. If you prefer no fruit chunks, puree the fruit first.

Kale Guacamole

DAIRY-FREE, GLUTEN-FREE, NUT-FREE, VEGAN

SERVES: 4 | **PREP TIME:** 10 minutes

This is a riff on the Simple Guacamole (page 41), but with a bit more flavor complexity, texture, and nutrition. Leafy greens are tricky to get into kids' diets (and into adults' diets, too). My hope is that this lovely side will help change that.

4 large kale leaves, thick stems and veins removed

¼ cup fresh cilantro leaves

2 ripe avocados, halved and pits removed, divided

½ teaspoon onion powder

¼ to ½ teaspoon sea salt

Pinch ground black pepper

Juice of 1 lime

1. Put the kale, cilantro leaves, and 1 avocado into a small food processor and puree until smooth. Periodically scrape down the sides of the processor bowl with a spatula.

2. In a medium bowl, mash the second avocado with a fork to your desired consistency. Add the onion powder, salt, pepper, and lime juice, as well as the kale and cilantro mixture. Stir well. Taste and adjust the seasoning as desired.

3. Serve baby 1 to 2 tablespoons on a plate or tray or preload a spoon and let them self-feed. Store leftovers in an airtight container in the refrigerator for up to 3 days. (Storing with the pit can help slow browning.)

TIP: For a smooth consistency or more of a spread, process the entire recipe. I *highly* recommend adding the salt on this one. Salt helps cut bitter flavors and makes the kale more enjoyable.

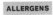

Chickpea Mash

DAIRY-FREE, GLUTEN-FREE, NUT-FREE, VEGAN

SERVES: 4 | **PREP TIME:** 5 minutes | **COOK TIME:** 10 minutes

Chickpeas are a great source of fiber and offer iron, zinc, and calcium. This recipe is intended to be a side dish, but for a main, you can double the recipe and put roasted vegetables on top. Please note that one of the cans of chickpeas should not be drained, as the liquid will be used in the recipe.

2 (15-ounce) cans no-salt-added chickpeas, 1 can drained and rinsed

2 teaspoons minced garlic

1 tablespoon gluten-free tamari

¼ to ½ teaspoon sea salt

¼ teaspoon ground black pepper

¼ cup green olives, pitted and diced

2 tablespoons chopped fresh parsley

½ teaspoon ground sumac

Juice of ½ lemon

Olive oil, for drizzling

1. In a medium saucepan over medium heat, combine the chickpeas and the liquid from 1 can of chickpeas along with the garlic and tamari. Simmer, mashing the chickpeas until a chunky mash has formed, 5 to 10 minutes.

2. Season with salt and pepper. Remove the pan from the heat. Add the olives, parsley, sumac, and lemon juice. Stir to mix evenly. Drizzle olive oil over the top.

3. Mash 2 tablespoons on a plate or tray, allow it cool, and serve it to baby on a plate or tray to eat with their hands or preload a spoon and let them self-feed. Store leftovers in an airtight container in the refrigerator for up to 4 days.

TIP: Try serving this side with the Spiced Turkey Meatballs (page 140) and Roasted Broccoli (page 46).

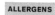

Applicious Overnight Oats

GLUTEN-FREE, NUT-FREE, VEGETARIAN

MAKES: About 1 cup | **PREP TIME:** 5 minutes, plus 4 hours to chill

Overnight oats allow you to prep breakfast the night before. This recipe uses the Stewed Cinnamon Ginger Apples to flavor and sweeten the oats. But, if you don't have that on hand—or the time to whip it up—try the Chia Seed Jam (page 68) or even some store-bought apple or pear sauce.

½ cup gluten-free oats

½ cup whole milk

1 tablespoon chia seeds

½ cup Stewed Cinnamon Ginger Apples (page 39) or store-bought applesauce

Maple syrup (optional)

1. Put the oats and milk into a mason jar or another storage container. Stir well.

2. Mix in the chia seeds and allow the mixture to sit for about 5 minutes to start thickening, then stir again.

3. Stir in the apples, then seal and refrigerate. Chill for 4 hours or overnight.

4. Taste and add a drizzle of maple syrup for more sweetness, if desired.

5. Before serving, stir well. Then serve baby 1 to 2 tablespoons on a plate or tray or preload a spoon and let them self-feed. Store leftovers in an airtight container in the refrigerator for up to 5 days.

TIP: For a looser oatmeal, stir in a bit more milk before serving. You can also warm up a serving before eating. Mashed banana, smashed peaches (canned or fresh), and berries are all delicious replacements for the apples.

Roasted Sweet and Salty Beets

GLUTEN-FREE, NUT-FREE, VEGETARIAN

SERVES: 4 | **PREP TIME:** 5 minutes | **COOK TIME:** 1 hour

Beets are naturally on the sweet side and are fun for babies to "paint" with on their tray, making them very inviting to little hands. This is a great time to strip baby down, unless you've got an outfit you're trying to ruin. Try this recipe for your next vegetable side dish.

2 large or 4 small beets, red, yellow, or a mix

1 to 2 tablespoons avocado oil

½ teaspoon sea salt, divided

1 tablespoon balsamic vinegar

1 tablespoon blue cheese, crumbled (optional)

1. Preheat the oven to 400°F.

2. Cut off the tip and stem ends of the beets to create a flat surface and remove any beet leaves. Place the beets on a large piece of foil.

3. Using your hands, coat the beets with the oil, then season them with ¼ teaspoon of salt. Wrap the foil around the beets and then place the foil packet on a baking sheet.

4. Bake the beets for 40 minutes, or until a fork glides through them with ease. If they're not there yet, continue baking and checking in 15-minute increments, up to 60 minutes.

5. Open the foil and allow the beets to cool until they are comfortable to handle. Using a peeler, remove the outer skin.

6. Cut the beets into ¼-inch strips, about the size of your pinky finger. Transfer the beets to a medium bowl and toss them with the vinegar, the remaining ¼ teaspoon of salt, and the blue cheese (if using).

7. Serve baby one or two strips, with a couple pieces of blue cheese, on a plate or tray to eat with their hands. Feel free to cut up the beet strips further for the rest of the family to eat with a fork. Store leftovers in an airtight container in the refrigerator for up to 4 days.

TIP: As baby gets older and develops a firm pincer grasp, you can cube the cooked beets and offer them that way, as well.

Broccoli and Sweet Potato Bites

GLUTEN-FREE, NUT-FREE

SERVES: 4 | **PREP TIME:** 10 minutes | **COOK TIME:** 25 minutes

These are a fun, simple side that comes together in no time if you use a food processor. And they're pretty pleasing to both child and adult palates. We love them alongside the Chicken Nuggets with a Boost (page 168) or the Chive and Cheese Dutch Baby (page 79), especially with a nice dipping sauce.

4 cups frozen broccoli, slightly thawed and squeezed to drain

½ large or 1 small sweet potato, cut into ½-inch-thick strips

1 cup shredded Parmesan cheese

1 large egg

2 teaspoons minced garlic

1 tablespoon ground flaxseed

¼ teaspoon sea salt

Pinch ground black pepper

1. Preheat the oven to 400°F. Line a large baking sheet with parchment paper.

2. In a food processor fitted with the shredding disk, feed the broccoli and then the sweet potato into the feeder tube, then transfer the shredded vegetables to a medium bowl.

3. Add the Parmesan, egg, garlic, flaxseed, salt, and pepper to the bowl and mix well to thoroughly combine.

4. Scoop up about 1 tablespoon of the mixture and form balls or 2-inch-long logs, then place them on the prepared baking sheet, leaving about 1 inch between each. Flatten slightly to create either patties or flattened sticks.

5. Bake for 10 minutes, then flip and bake another 10 to 15 minutes, or until the patties start to brown. Feel free to bake longer for an even softer texture.

6. Remove the patties from the pan and allow them to cool for about 5 minutes.

7. Serve baby one or two bites on a plate or tray to eat with their hands. Store leftovers in an airtight container in the refrigerator for up to 4 days. Reheat in the oven for 5 to 10 minutes until warmed through.

Black Lentils with Squash and Herbs

DAIRY-FREE, GLUTEN-FREE, NUT-FREE, VEGAN

SERVES: 4+ | **PREP TIME:** 15 minutes | **COOK TIME:** 20 minutes

Lentils are a great inexpensive protein and fiber option and are super baby-friendly. I recommend black lentils for the best consistency. Add a fried egg, ball of mozzarella, or grilled chicken on top for a more filling meal. This can be eaten warm or at room temperature. Lentils can also be soaked overnight to increase digestibility.

3 cups water

1½ cups dried black lentils

7 tablespoons olive oil, divided

2 cups finely diced skin-on Delicata squash

1 small sweet onion, diced

1 teaspoon dried thyme

½ teaspoon sea salt, divided

Pinch ground black pepper

2 teaspoons minced garlic

1 cup fresh basil, finely sliced

1 tablespoon apple cider vinegar

2 teaspoons Dijon mustard

1. In a medium saucepan, combine the water and lentils and bring them to a boil over high heat. Turn down the heat to low and simmer the lentils for about 20 minutes, or until tender. Drain.

2. While the lentils cook, heat a large pan over medium heat and add 1 tablespoon of olive oil. Add the squash, onion, thyme, ¼ teaspoon of salt, and the pepper, stirring until slightly browned and tender, about 10 minutes.

3. Add the garlic and cook for 1 minute more. Add the cooked lentils and mix well. Turn off the heat and add the basil, vinegar, mustard, and remaining 6 tablespoons of olive oil. Stir thoroughly to combine. Taste and adjust the seasoning as desired.

4. Let 1 to 2 tablespoons cool, then serve to baby on a plate or tray to eat with their hands or preload a spoon and let them self-feed. Store leftovers in an airtight container in the refrigerator for up to 5 days.

Coconut Curried Kidney Beans

DAIRY-FREE, GLUTEN-FREE, VEGAN

SERVES: 4+ | **PREP TIME:** 10 minutes | **COOK TIME:** 20 minutes

This is a simple, flavorful dish that can be served as is, or with tofu, shrimp, or chicken for a more robust meal. I recommend starting with 1 tablespoon of red curry paste and then increasing to your desired heat level.

2 tablespoons coconut oil

1 small sweet onion, diced

1 (1-inch) piece fresh ginger, peeled and finely grated (about 1 tablespoon)

1 tablespoon minced garlic

1 red bell pepper, diced

1 to 2 tablespoons Thai red curry paste

1 tablespoon tomato paste

1 (14-ounce) can full-fat coconut milk

Pinch sea salt

2 (15-ounce) cans no-salt-added kidney beans, drained and rinsed

1. In a medium saucepan, melt the coconut oil over medium-high heat. Add the onion, ginger, and garlic and sauté for 1 to 2 minutes, or until fragrant.

2. Add the bell pepper and stir for 1 minute. Turn down the heat to medium, then mix in the curry paste and tomato paste, stirring until everything is well coated. Then add the coconut milk and salt and stir.

3. Simmer for 15 minutes, then add the beans and simmer for another 2 minutes.

4. Using a slotted spoon, scoop out 2 tablespoons of beans, allow them to cool, then serve them to baby in a bowl or on their tray to eat with their hands. Store leftovers in an airtight container in the refrigerator for up to 4 days.

TIP: Try serving this with the Basic Cauliflower Rice (page 97) or store-bought riced cauliflower. You can add other vegetables that are chopped small and cooked until tender, such as broccoli, cauliflower, or green beans.

ALLERGENS

Chive and Cheese Dutch Baby

GLUTEN-FREE, NUT-FREE, VEGETARIAN

SERVES: 4 | **PREP TIME:** 5 minutes | **COOK TIME:** 15 minutes

Not familiar with a Dutch baby? Neither was I! In fact, this recipe came about *while* I was working on this book and trying to throw something together for dinner one night. My four-year-old announced that she would "eat this all day" and it should "absolutely, definitely" be in the book. So, here it is!

4 large eggs

⅔ cup gluten-free flour mix

⅔ cup whole milk

¼ to ½ teaspoon sea salt

¼ teaspoon ground black pepper

2 tablespoons finely diced fresh chives

½ cup shredded sharp cheddar cheese

3 tablespoons unsalted butter

1. Preheat the oven to 450°F.

2. In a medium bowl, whisk together the eggs, flour, and milk until smooth. Whisk in the salt and pepper, then gently stir in the chives and cheese.

3. In a large oven-safe skillet, melt the butter over medium heat. Turn off the heat and swirl the butter around to coat the entire pan and sides. Pour in the batter. Bake for 12 to 15 minutes, or until the Dutch baby starts to puff and the edges are starting to turn golden brown.

4. Cut a section of the Dutch baby into thin strips and allow them to cool for baby. Serve baby the strips on a plate or tray to eat with their hands. Store leftovers in an airtight container in the refrigerator for up to 4 days.

TIP: Feel free to change up the type of cheese, dice up different vegetables to mix in, or sauté mushrooms, onion, or leeks to put on top of the finished Dutch baby.

Beef and Bean Chili

DAIRY-FREE, GLUTEN-FREE, NUT-FREE
SERVES: 4+ | **PREP TIME:** 15 minutes | **COOK TIME:** 40 minutes

Chili is a great option for new eaters and the whole family, and a perfect dish in which to hide liver. You can make this meat-free, but if you do so, I recommend adding some diced spinach to increase the iron content. Please note that some brands of Worcestershire sauce may contain soy sauce, which often contains gluten. If you need this dish to be gluten-free, be sure to read the label.

1 tablespoon avocado oil

1 small yellow onion, diced

1 large bell pepper, any color, diced

3 teaspoons minced garlic

1 pound ground beef, preferably grass-fed

½ pound sausage (Italian, sweet, or spicy)

3 ounces chicken liver, finely diced (optional)

1 tablespoon cumin

2 teaspoons smoked paprika

1 teaspoon dried oregano

2 teaspoons gluten-free Worcestershire sauce

2 (28-ounce) cans tomato puree or sauce

2 (15-ounce) cans no-salt-added beans (kidney, pinto, black beans, or a combination), rinsed and drained

1. In a large stockpot, heat the oil over medium heat. Add the onion and bell pepper and sauté until soft, about 5 minutes. Stir in the garlic and cook for another minute, or until fragrant.

2. Add the beef, sausage, and liver (if using), and cook for about 10 minutes, stirring and breaking up the meat, until the meat has browned.

3. Add the cumin, paprika, oregano, and Worcestershire sauce and stir well. Then mix in the tomato puree and beans.

4. Cover and bring the chili to a boil. Stir, then turn down the heat to low and simmer for at least 10 minutes, stirring occasionally to prevent sticking. (If you'd like a thicker chili, continue cooking without a lid until your desired thickness is reached.)

5. Using a slotted spoon, scoop out 2 tablespoons of chili, allow it to cool, and serve it to baby in a bowl or on their tray to eat with their hands or practice using a spoon. Store leftovers in an airtight container in the refrigerator for up to 4 days or in the freezer for about 5 months.

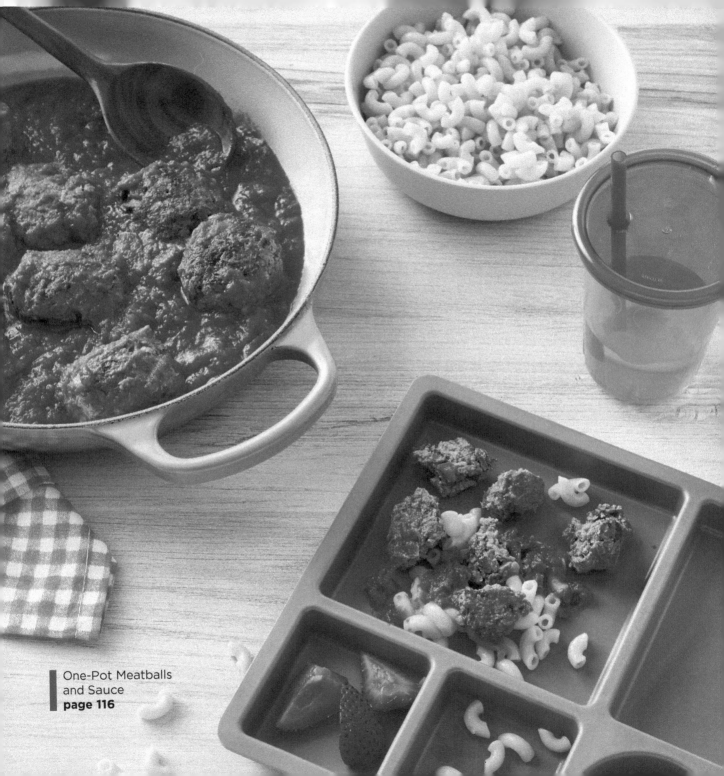

One-Pot Meatballs
and Sauce
page 116

CHAPTER 5

The More (Food), the Merrier (9 to 12 Months)

Velvety Vanilla Smoothie

GLUTEN-FREE, VEGETARIAN

MAKES: 8 ounces | **PREP TIME:** 10 minutes

By 9 to 12 months, most little ones are getting pretty good with straws and pouches. This smoothie is a great option for a reusable pouch or a straw cup (a regular straw or thicker straw is a better option than a thin-straw toddler cup, as the smoothie will be a bit too thick for a tiny straw). You can serve the smoothie to baby as a simple breakfast or a great snack on the go.

1 cup whole milk

½ avocado

2 big handfuls fresh spinach

2 teaspoons vanilla extract, plus more as needed

½ teaspoon almond extract, plus more as needed (optional)

1 to 2 tablespoons maple syrup or Date Paste (page 40)

Pinch sea salt

3 or 4 ice cubes

1. Put the milk, avocado, spinach, vanilla, almond extract (if using), maple syrup, and salt into a blender and blend until very smooth.

2. Taste and adjust sweetness and the vanilla and almond flavors as desired. Add the ice cubes and blend again until the ice is in small pieces.

3. Pour 2 to 4 ounces into a cup with a straw or reusable pouch for baby to enjoy. Pour leftovers into ice pop molds and store in the freezer for up to 1 month.

TIP: For a dairy-free option, Ripple milk, Homemade Almond Milk (page 62), or Homemade Oat Milk (page 64) are great. For a chocolate twist, reduce the vanilla to 1 teaspoon and add 1 tablespoon cocoa powder.

Chamomile Apple Ginger Gelatin

DAIRY-FREE, GLUTEN-FREE, NUT-FREE

MAKES: About 32 strips | **PREP TIME:** 10 minutes, plus 2 hours to chill |
COOK TIME: 10 minutes

A wonderful anytime snack, these gelatin strips are made with gelatin from grass-fed cows, a great source of protein and gut-healing amino acids. The chamomile and ginger provide digestive support and ease tummy troubles.

6 ounces water

1 bag chamomile tea

1 (1-inch) piece fresh ginger, coarsely chopped

1¼ cup apple juice at room temperature, divided

1 tablespoon gelatin from grass-fed cows

1. Line an 8-by-8-inch pan with parchment paper. In a small saucepan over high heat, bring the water, chamomile, and ginger to a boil. Boil for about 3 minutes.

2. Meanwhile, pour ½ cup of the juice into a large mixing bowl. Sprinkle the gelatin over it and whisk vigorously. Let it sit for 2 minutes to thicken.

3. Remove the ginger and tea bag from the water and pour the liquid slowly into the large mixing bowl, whisking continuously, until the mixture is completely smooth. Whisk in the remaining ¾ cup juice, then pour the liquid into the prepared pan. Refrigerate for at least 2 hours, or until set.

4. Cut the gelatin into 2-inch-by-1-inch strips and serve baby one strip at a time on a plate or tray to eat with their hands. Store leftovers in an airtight container in the refrigerator for up to 7 days.

TIP: For a more gummy-like texture for older children, add 1 to 2 tablespoons more of gelatin and pour the liquid into molds to set.

Prune Bars

DAIRY-FREE, GLUTEN-FREE

MAKES: 16 bars | **PREP TIME:** 15 minutes | **CHILL TIME:** 1 hour

Starting solids can sometimes be quite the transition for your little one's digestive system. Constipation or shifts in bowel movements are common. These bars were an absolute miracle for our oldest daughter. She was tube-fed the first year of her life, and weaning her off the tube was quite the experience, especially because she wasn't keen on fluids at first. These bars help keep kids regular and also provide some incredible nutrition.

½ cup walnuts

¼ cup pumpkin seeds

1 cup pitted prunes, chopped

3 tablespoons cocoa powder

2 tablespoons chia seeds

2 tablespoons hemp seeds

2 tablespoons all-natural creamy nut butter of choice

2 tablespoons coconut oil, melted

2 tablespoons collagen powder (optional)

2 tablespoons finely ground flaxseed, divided

1. Line a 4-inch-by-8-inch loaf pan with parchment paper.

2. Put the walnuts and pumpkin seeds in a food processor and pulse them until they are finely ground. Add the prunes, cocoa powder, chia seeds, hemp seeds, and nut butter. Pulse until well combined. Add the coconut oil and collagen (if using) and pulse until the mixture forms a ball that holds together.

3. Sprinkle half the ground flaxseed evenly along the bottom of the lined pan. Transfer the prune mixture into the prepared pan and press until flat.

4. Sprinkle the remaining flaxseed evenly over the top. Refrigerate for 1 hour, then lift the parchment paper out of the pan and transfer it to the cutting board.

5. Cut into 2-inch-by-1-inch bars. Serve baby one bar at a time on a plate or tray to eat with their hands. Store leftovers in an airtight container, separating layers of bars with parchment paper, in the refrigerator for up to 5 days.

TIP: Ground flaxseed itself can be a great bathroom helper. Sprinkle it on top of oatmeal or yogurt. Feel free to use all pumpkin seeds in place of the walnuts, and tahini or sunflower seed butter for a nut-free option.

Banana Soft-Serve

DAIRY-FREE, GLUTEN-FREE, VEGAN

MAKES: About 1 cup | **PREP TIME:** 10 minutes

Ice cream is such a yummy treat, but it's not ideal for a baby. This is a simple and fun way to do "ice cream" for the whole family. Go slow with adding the liquid. If you add too much liquid too fast, you'll end up with a frozen soup. Expect it to look like really bad Dippin' Dots at first, but when you keep going slowly, it will turn into a fluffy soft-serve.

1 frozen banana, cut into ½- to 1-inch chunks

1 tablespoon all-natural creamy peanut butter (optional)

Handful of spinach (optional)

¼ to ½ cup additional frozen fruit (optional)

2 tablespoons cocoa powder (optional)

Up to ¼ cup full-fat coconut milk

1. Put the frozen banana and your choice of the optional ingredients into a food processor. Begin to pulse the ingredients until rice-like grains form. Continue pulsing, slowly drizzling in coconut milk, as needed, to keep things moving. Pulse until light and fluffy.

2. Serve baby 2 to 4 tablespoons in a bowl with a spoon and let them self-feed. Pour leftovers into ice pop molds and store in the freezer for up to 2 weeks.

TIP: Try this with a different base fruit (such as frozen strawberries, frozen pineapple, or frozen peaches) and add toppings (chia seeds, chopped nuts, chocolate chips, chopped fruit, Dairy-Free Whipped Cream [page 59] or sprinkles).

Mochi Corn Bread Muffins

GLUTEN-FREE, NUT-FREE, VEGETARIAN

MAKES: 10 regular or 24 mini muffins | **PREP TIME:** 10 minutes | **COOK TIME:** 30 minutes

This recipe, made with sticky rice flour, is gluten-free and has a super-fun texture. You can find mochiko flour at a specialty store, Asian grocery store, or on Amazon. Make sure you get the *sweet rice* flour, not regular rice flour.

1 cup mochiko sweet rice flour

1 cup finely ground cornmeal

2 teaspoons baking powder

Pinch salt

1¼ cup whole milk

⅓ cup avocado oil

3 to 4 tablespoons maple syrup

1 large egg

1. Preheat the oven to 350°F. Grease a muffin tin (regular or mini) or use cupcake liners.

2. In a large bowl, whisk together all the ingredients until a smooth batter forms. Fill each muffin cup nearly to the top.

3. Bake for about 25 minutes for regular muffins or 12 minutes for mini muffins. The muffins will be done when a toothpick inserted into the center comes out clean. Cool for 5 to 10 minutes in the pan, then transfer to a cooling rack.

4. Serve large muffins cut up into strips or mini muffins cut into quarters on a plate or tray for baby to eat with their hands. Store leftovers in an airtight container on the counter for up to 3 days, or freeze the muffins on a cookie sheet, then transfer to an airtight container and store in the freezer for up to 3 months.

TIP: For an 8-by-8-inch pan, line with parchment paper and bake for about 30 minutes, then cut into strips or squares.

Double Chocolate Chip Veggie Muffins

DAIRY-FREE, GLUTEN-FREE, NUT-FREE

MAKES: 12 regular or 30 mini muffins | **PREP TIME:** 15 minutes | **COOK TIME:** 20 minutes

Packed with vegetables and naturally sweetened with dates, these muffins are a favorite in our house. Be sure to use dairy-free chocolate chips if you need this recipe to be dairy-free.

1 cup sweet potato, cooked and chopped into 1-inch chunks (about 2 small sweet potatoes)

2 to 3 big handfuls of fresh spinach (about half of a 5-ounce bag)

6 to 8 large Medjool dates, pitted and soaked in hot water for 10 minutes, soaking liquid reserved

¼ cup avocado oil

3 large eggs

1 teaspoon vanilla extract

1 to 2 heaping tablespoons collagen powder (optional)

¾ cup cocoa powder

1 teaspoon baking soda

Pinch sea salt

2 tablespoons maple syrup (optional)

1 cup dairy-free dark chocolate chips (mini or regular)

1. Preheat the oven to 350°F. Grease a muffin tin (regular or mini) or use cupcake liners.

2. Put the sweet potato, spinach, dates, oil, eggs, and vanilla into a blender or food processor and blend until smooth. If the batter is too thick, slowly drizzle in the reserved date soaking water.

3. Add the collagen powder (if using), cocoa powder, baking soda, and salt and blend until just combined. Taste and add maple syrup, if desired. Toss in chocolate chips and blend briefly.

4. Fill each muffin cup about three-quarters full. Bake for 15 to 20 minutes, or until a toothpick inserted in the center comes out clean. Cool for 5 to 10 minutes in the pan, then transfer to a cooling rack to cool completely.

5. Serve large muffins cut up into strips or mini muffins cut into quarters on a plate or tray for baby to eat with their hands. Store leftovers in an airtight container in the refrigerator for up to 5 days or freeze the muffins on a cookie sheet, then transfer to an airtight container and store in the freezer for up to 3 months.

Blueberry Almond Muffins

DAIRY-FREE, GLUTEN-FREE, VEGETARIAN
MAKES: 10 regular or 30 mini muffins | **PREP TIME:** 15 minutes | **COOK TIME:** 25 minutes

These muffins are protein-packed and a wonderfully easy finger food for kiddos. Bonus? They're delicious *and* nutrient-rich, unlike most ready-made baked goods. If you use frozen berries, be sure to let them thaw in a strainer so the extra juices can drain a bit, but do *not* rinse.

2 cups almond flour

3 large eggs

1 medium sweet potato, cooked, peeled, and mashed

3 tablespoons maple syrup or Date Paste (page 40)

1 tablespoon ground flaxseed

1 teaspoon baking powder

¼ teaspoon sea salt

1 teaspoon vanilla extract

½ teaspoon almond extract (optional)

1 cup fresh or frozen blueberries (thawed and drained if frozen)

1. Preheat the oven to 350°F. Grease a muffin tin (regular or mini) or use cupcake liners.

2. In a large bowl, combine the flour, eggs, sweet potato, maple syrup, flaxseed, baking powder, salt, vanilla, and almond extract (if using). Stir until the batter is fairly smooth. Gently fold in the blueberries.

3. Fill each muffin cup nearly to the top.

4. Bake for about 25 minutes for regular muffins or 15 to 20 minutes for mini muffins. The muffins will be done when the tops are golden and a toothpick inserted into the center comes out clean. Cool for 5 to 10 minutes in the pan, then transfer to a cooling rack to cool completely.

5. Serve large muffins cut up into strips or mini muffins cut into quarters on a plate or tray for baby to eat with their hands. Store leftovers in an airtight container in the refrigerator for up to 5 days or freeze the muffins on a cookie sheet, then transfer to an airtight container and store in the freezer for up to 3 months.

Zucchini Bread Baked Oatmeal

GLUTEN-FREE, NUT-FREE, VEGETARIAN
SERVES: 4 | **PREP TIME:** 15 minutes | **COOK TIME:** 35 minutes

Baked oatmeal is such a nice, warm start to the day and allows you to drink your coffee, jump in the shower, or snuggle with baby while it bakes. I love how hands-off it is, and sneaking vegetables in for breakfast is always a win in my book. Remember to choose gluten-free oats if you want this to be gluten-free.

2 cups gluten-free oats

1 small zucchini, finely shredded and squeezed to remove excess liquid

1 teaspoon ground cinnamon

¼ teaspoon ground nutmeg

1 cup whole milk

2 large eggs

⅓ cup maple syrup or Date Paste (page 40)

¼ cup avocado oil

1 teaspoon vanilla extract

1. Preheat the oven to 350°F. Line an 8-by-8-inch pan with parchment paper.

2. In a large mixing bowl, mix together all the ingredients until well combined. Pour the batter into the prepared baking pan.

3. Bake for 30 to 35 minutes, or until the center is set and the edges are just starting to brown. Allow to cool for 5 minutes, then cut into squares.

4. Cut one square into strips and serve to baby on a plate or tray to eat with their hands. Store leftovers in an airtight container in the refrigerator for 5 days.

TIP: For a protein boost, add a few scoops of collagen powder. Serve with some Dairy-Free Whipped Cream (page 59).

Blueberry Dutch Baby

GLUTEN-FREE, NUT-FREE, VEGETARIAN

SERVES: 4 | **PREP TIME:** 10 minutes | **COOK TIME:** 15 minutes

I love pancakes for breakfast, but I hate standing over the stove dishing out pancakes as fast as the kids devour them. Enter the Blueberry Dutch Baby. It's like a baked blueberry pancake that's ready for everyone at the same time. For a complete meal, serve with sides or double the recipe and make two pans' worth.

4 large eggs

⅔ cup gluten-free flour mix

⅔ cup whole milk

1 tablespoon maple syrup

1 teaspoon vanilla extract

½ cup fresh or frozen small blueberries (thawed and drained if frozen)

3 tablespoons unsalted butter

1. Preheat the oven to 450°F.

2. In a medium bowl, whisk together the eggs, flour, milk, maple syrup, and vanilla until smooth. Then gently fold in the blueberries.

3. In a large skillet, melt the butter over medium heat. Remove the pan from the heat, turn off the stove, and swirl the butter around to coat the entire pan and sides. Pour the batter into the pan. Bake for 12 to 15 minutes, or until the Dutch baby starts to puff and the edges are starting to turn golden brown.

4. Cut a section of the Dutch baby into thin strips and allow them to cool. Serve baby the cooled strips on a plate or tray to eat with their hands. Store leftovers in an airtight container in the refrigerator for up to 4 days.

TIP: For a chocolaty spin, omit 2 to 4 tablespoons of flour and replace it with cocoa powder.

Tangy and Sweet Shredded Brussels Sprouts

DAIRY-FREE, GLUTEN-FREE, NUT-FREE, VEGAN
SERVES: 4 | **PREP TIME:** 10 minutes | **COOK TIME:** 25 minutes

Shredded Brussels sprouts are a bit more advanced in texture, but thanks to the fine shred and cooking, they tend to be manageable at this stage. The sweet and tangy flavors make this often-rejected vegetable much more interesting.

1 pound Brussels sprouts, thick ends removed and very finely shredded

1 tablespoon avocado oil

Maple syrup, for drizzling

1 heaping teaspoon minced garlic

1 teaspoon Dijon mustard

½ teaspoon sea salt

Pinch ground black pepper

1. Preheat the oven to 425°F. Line a large baking sheet with parchment paper.

2. Put the Brussels sprouts in a large bowl, then add the remaining ingredients and toss to thoroughly coat the Brussels sprouts. Transfer the Brussels sprouts to the prepared sheet and spread them out in a thin layer.

3. Bake for 15 minutes, then toss and bake for another 5 to 10 minutes, or until they're tender and starting to brown.

4. Let a 1- to 2-tablespoon portion cool, then serve it to baby on a plate or tray to eat with their hands or practice using a spoon. Store leftovers in an airtight container in the refrigerator for up to 3 days.

Basic Cauliflower Rice

DAIRY-FREE, GLUTEN-FREE, NUT-FREE, VEGAN

SERVES: 4+ | **PREP TIME:** 10 minutes | **COOK TIME:** 10 minutes

Cauliflower rice is one of my favorite tricks. It's an easy, versatile way to incorporate more vegetables, fiber, and nutrients into meals. This is the most basic version, but you can absolutely spice it up just like you would regular rice.

1 head cauliflower, cut into quarters
1 tablespoon avocado oil

Sea salt

1. One quarter at a time, break up the cauliflower into smaller florets and then pulse in a food processor to your desired size. Quinoa-size bits are great for new eaters.

2. Once all the cauliflower is processed, put it in a large skillet and drizzle the oil over it. Cook over medium-high heat for 5 minutes, stirring periodically, until the cauliflower starts to soften.

3. Season with salt. Continue cooking to your desired consistency, 2 to 5 minutes more for al dente, and 5 minutes or more for a softer option.

4. Let 1 to 2 tablespoons cool for baby, then serve it on a plate or tray for them to eat with their hands or practice using a spoon. Store leftovers in an airtight container in the refrigerator for up to 5 days.

TIP: Raw cauliflower rice can be frozen for up to a month in an airtight container. You can also boil the rice in water or bake it in the oven. No food processor? Use a cheese grater or buy the pre-riced cauliflower from the store, often found either in the freezer section or in the produce section.

Gazpacho

DAIRY-FREE, GLUTEN-FREE, NUT-FREE, VEGAN

SERVES: 4 | **PREP TIME:** 10 minutes, plus 2 hours to cool

This chilled soup is a wonderful way to use up fresh summer tomatoes, especially those that might seem "imperfect." You can use one color or kind of tomato or a mix of heirloom varieties for more complex flavor and color. Summer farmers' markets will likely have many types to choose from.

8 medium to large very ripe tomatoes, halved, divided

1 large bell pepper, any color, seeded and cut into rough strips

1 small cucumber, cut into rough chunks

¼ to ⅓ cup diced scallions, white and green parts

½ jalapeño pepper, seeded and finely diced

1 heaping teaspoon minced garlic

Juice of 1 lime

2 tablespoons olive oil

1 to 2 tablespoons white vinegar

2 teaspoons dried parsley

1 teaspoon ground cumin

1 teaspoon dried basil

½ teaspoon sea salt

Pinch ground black pepper

1. Put 4 or 5 tomatoes in a blender and blend until smooth. Pour the pureed tomatoes into a large bowl.

2. Put the remaining 3 or 4 tomatoes, the bell pepper, cucumber, scallions, jalapeño, garlic, lime juice, olive oil, and vinegar into the blender and pulse until the vegetables are just slightly chunky. Pour this mixture into the large bowl of blended tomatoes.

3. Stir in the parsley, cumin, basil, salt, and pepper. Taste and adjust the seasoning as desired. Chill for at least 2 hours.

4. Serve baby 2 to 4 tablespoons of the soup in a bowl with a spoon and let them self-feed. Store leftovers in an airtight container in the refrigerator for up to 5 days.

TIP: As baby gets older, you can let the vegetables be chunkier, but for new eaters, I recommend a smoother consistency. This soup can be served with a large straw or reusable pouch if you make it completely smooth.

Apple Arugula Breakfast Sausage

DAIRY-FREE, GLUTEN-FREE, NUT-FREE

SERVES: 4 | **PREP TIME:** 10 minutes | **COOK TIME:** 20 minutes

Sausage can be a great way to get protein for breakfast, but store-bought sausage tends to be little more than meat, fat, and a couple of spices. Plus, sausage links in a casing need to be very carefully cut to avoid becoming a choking hazard. This homemade option comes together quickly and can be made into patties or cooked as is and broken up into crumbles to add to quiche or scrambled eggs or even an evening pasta dish.

1 pound ground pork

½ large sweet onion, finely diced

1 medium green apple, peeled and shredded

1 cup fresh arugula, finely chopped

1 teaspoon dried thyme

1 teaspoon smoked paprika

½ teaspoon sea salt

Pinch ground black pepper

1 to 2 tablespoons avocado oil, divided

1. Line a platter with paper towels.

2. In a large bowl, mix together the pork, onion, apple, arugula, thyme, paprika, salt, and pepper until well combined.

3. Scooping 1 to 2 tablespoons of sausage into your hands at a time, form ½-inch-thick patties. Place them on a large plate and set aside.

4. In a large cast-iron skillet, heat the oil over medium heat. Put about 5 of the patties into the skillet, being careful not to overcrowd the pan. Cook for about 4 minutes, or until the patties start to brown, then flip and cook for another 3 to 4 minutes, or until both sides are browned and the internal temperature reaches 165°F. Transfer to the prepared platter. Repeat steps 3 and 4 with the remaining meat mixture.

5. Let a patty cool, then serve it to baby whole or cut into finger-size strips on a plate or tray to eat with their hands. Store leftovers in an airtight container in the refrigerator for up to 4 days.

Barbecue Baked Tofu

DAIRY-FREE, GLUTEN-FREE, NUT-FREE, VEGAN

SERVES: 4 | **PREP TIME:** 5 minutes, plus 30 minutes to rest | **COOK TIME:** 30 minutes

Tofu can be a great protein option for new eaters. The texture tends to be much easier than most protein sources and it pairs well with many flavor combinations. Feel free to eat the leftovers cold, straight from the refrigerator. You can add a flavor twist by mixing peanut butter or almond butter into the barbecue sauce before tossing.

2 (14-ounce) blocks extra-firm tofu

2 tablespoons toasted sesame seed oil

4 tablespoons barbecue sauce, divided (check for gluten-free if needed)

1. Place the tofu on its long edge and carefully cut it in half so there are two thinner tofu rectangles. Repeat with the second block.

2. Place the four large rectangles of tofu on top of a clean kitchen towel or several layers of paper towels on a cutting board. Cover with the other half of the towel or additional paper towels. Place another cutting board on top and place something heavy, like a large soup pot, on top of the second cutting board. Let the tofu sit for 30 minutes.

3. Preheat the oven to 400°F. Line a large baking sheet with parchment paper.

4. Remove the towels and place the tofu on a cutting board and cut it into ½-inch strips. Gently transfer the strips to a large bowl and add the oil and 2 tablespoons of barbecue sauce. Toss gently to coat.

5. Place the strips on the prepared baking sheet, leaving ½ to 1 inch between strips. Bake for 15 minutes, flip, then bake for another 10 to 15 minutes, or until the tofu starts to brown.

6. Place the baked tofu back in the large bowl and toss with the remaining 2 tablespoons of barbecue sauce.

7. Let 1 to 2 strips cool, then serve baby the strips on a plate or tray to eat with their hands. Store leftovers in an airtight container in the refrigerator for up to 4 days.

Canned Salmon Cakes

DAIRY-FREE, GLUTEN-FREE, NUT-FREE

SERVES: 4 | **PREP TIME:** 10 minutes | **COOK TIME:** 15 minutes

These salmon cakes make adding fish to your baby's diet a cinch. I love using canned fish and seafood, as it tends to be less expensive. Cans of salmon come in different amounts, hence the range listed in the ingredients. If you have leftover Grilled Salmon (page 55), you can use that instead of the canned, or a combination of the two.

3 small to medium red potatoes, quartered

12 to 16 ounces canned salmon

1 small bell pepper, any color, diced

½ large yellow onion, finely diced

¼ cup chopped fresh parsley, or 2 tablespoons dried parsley

1 large egg

Juice of ½ lemon

2 teaspoons yellow mustard

1 tablespoon ground flaxseed

½ teaspoon sea salt

Pinch ground black pepper

1. Put the potatoes in a small stockpot, cover them with water, and bring to a boil over medium-high heat. Boil the potatoes for about 10 minutes, or until easily pierced with a fork. Drain and set aside to cool.

2. Meanwhile, preheat the oven to 350°F. Line a large baking sheet with parchment paper.

3. In a large bowl, combine the salmon, bell pepper, onion, parsley, egg, lemon juice, mustard, flaxseed, salt, and pepper and mix well.

4. Mash the potatoes, then stir them into the salmon mixture.

5. Scoop ¼ cup of the salmon mixture at a time and place each scoop on the prepared baking sheet, spacing the cakes about 2 inches apart.

6. Bake for 12 to 14 minutes, or until the edges are just starting to brown, then broil for 2 to 3 minutes until browned. (Keep an eye on them so they don't burn.)

7. Let a salmon cake cool, then cut it into halves or quarters and serve to baby on a plate or tray to eat with their hands or a fork. Store leftovers in an airtight container in the refrigerator for up to 4 days.

Curry Quinoa Bowl

DAIRY-FREE, GLUTEN-FREE, NUT-FREE

SERVES: 4 | **PREP TIME:** 15 minutes | **COOK TIME:** 15 minutes

This quinoa bowl is an adaptable recipe that's delicious warm or cold. You can use different vegetables or add proteins, such as Barbecue Baked Tofu (page 102).

1½ cups dry quinoa

3 cups Slow Cooker Bone Broth (page 36), store-bought broth, or water

4 tablespoons olive oil

3 tablespoons apple cider vinegar

1 to 2 tablespoons maple syrup

2 teaspoons minced garlic

1 tablespoon curry powder

¼ teaspoon sea salt

1 (15-ounce) can no-salt-added black beans, drained and rinsed

1 bell pepper, any color, seeded and finely chopped

2 scallions, white and green parts, very thinly sliced

1 orange, peeled and chopped

1. In a medium stockpot over high heat, combine the quinoa and broth. Bring the broth to a boil, then turn down the heat to low and simmer for 15 minutes, or until the liquid is absorbed.

2. Meanwhile, make the dressing. In a small bowl, whisk together the olive oil, vinegar, maple syrup, garlic, curry powder, and salt.

3. When the quinoa is cooked, transfer it to a large mixing bowl. Add the remaining ingredients, mix until well combined, then toss with the dressing.

4. Let 2 to 4 tablespoons cool, then serve to baby on a plate or in a bowl. Store leftovers in an airtight container in the refrigerator for up to 5 days.

Simple Crab Cakes

DAIRY-FREE, GLUTEN-FREE, NUT-FREE
SERVES: 4 | **PREP TIME:** 5 minutes | **COOK TIME:** 10 minutes

We love these with a side salad and some Roasted Asparagus Spears (page 56). The lump crabmeat is typically found in the refrigerated seafood section of the grocery store. You can use claw meat instead of lump, but the lump is sweeter, and the claw meat needs to be checked for any small shell shards.

1 pound jumbo lump crabmeat
3 to 4 tablespoons mayonnaise
Juice of ½ lemon

1 to 2 teaspoons Old Bay seasoning
¼ teaspoon ground black pepper

1. Preheat the oven to 350°F. Line a large baking sheet with parchment paper.

2. In a large bowl, mix all the ingredients together gently. Taste and adjust the seasoning as desired.

3. Gently form four large crab cakes and place them on the prepared baking sheet, 2 inches apart. Bake for about 8 minutes, or until the crab cakes just start to brown at the edges, then broil for an additional minute to add some color to the top of the crab cake. (Keep an eye on them so they don't burn.)

4. Let a crab cake cool, then cut it into halves or in quarters and serve to baby on a plate or tray to eat with their hands or a fork. Store leftovers in an airtight container in the refrigerator for up to 4 days.

Not Your Grandma's Chicken Soup

DAIRY-FREE, GLUTEN-FREE, NUT-FREE

SERVES: 6+ | **PREP TIME:** 15 minutes | **COOK TIME:** 6 hours

This soup is perfect for a cold winter evening, especially if anyone in the family is feeling under the weather. It's rich in collagen from bone broth, and rich in protein, vitamins, and minerals from the vegetables. With the added immune support from the ginger, this is food as medicine at its best. We generally cook a whole chicken in the slow cooker the day before or throughout the day, but a rotisserie chicken is a great option, too.

3 tablespoons avocado oil

8 ounces white button mushrooms, diced

3 small red potatoes, chopped into ¼-inch chunks

1 large sweet onion, diced

2 large leeks, thinly sliced

2 celery stalks, finely diced

1 large carrot, finely diced

2 teaspoons minced garlic

¼ teaspoon sea salt

Pinch ground black pepper

4 cups Slow Cooker Bone Broth (page 36) or store-bought bone broth, divided

1 (5-ounce) bag baby spinach

1-inch piece fresh ginger, peeled

Meat from 1 whole chicken, cooked and chopped (about 3 cups)

Juice of 1 lemon

1. In a large stockpot, heat the oil over medium-high heat. Add the mushrooms, potatoes, onion, leeks, celery, carrot, garlic, salt, and pepper. Cook, stirring occasionally, for about 10 minutes, or until the vegetables start to soften.

2. Meanwhile, put 2 cups of the broth, the spinach, and ginger in a blender and blend until smooth, 1 to 2 minutes.

3. When the vegetables are ready, add the spinach and ginger broth and remaining 2 cups of bone broth to the stockpot and bring them to a simmer. Add the chicken, stir, and continue to simmer, covered, for at least 20 minutes, or until the carrots and potatoes can be easily pierced with a fork. Stir in the lemon juice.

4. Using a slotted spoon, scoop out 2 to 4 tablespoons of chicken and vegetables into a bowl, let cool, then serve it to baby to eat with their hands or a spoon. Store leftovers in an airtight container in the refrigerator for up to 4 days or in the freezer for up to 3 months.

TIP: Toss the chicken bones and skin, as well as any vegetable "trimmings," back into the slow cooker to make a batch of the Slow Cooker Bone Broth (page 36).

White Chicken Chili

GLUTEN-FREE, NUT-FREE

SERVES: 4+ | **PREP TIME:** 15 minutes | **COOK TIME:** 30 minutes

This chicken chili is a favorite dinner, especially with the Mochi Corn Bread Muffins (page 89). We usually do a whole chicken in the slow cooker all day, then pull the meat off for the soup in the evening, or use a store-bought rotisserie chicken in a pinch.

2 tablespoons avocado oil

1 small yellow onion, finely chopped

1 celery stalk, finely diced

1 large carrot, finely diced

4 ounces white button mushrooms, finely chopped

1 heaping teaspoon minced garlic

2 teaspoons ground cumin

1 teaspoon smoked paprika

½ teaspoon sea salt

Pinch cayenne (optional)

Pinch ground black pepper

2 (15-ounce) cans no-salt-added white kidney beans, rinsed and drained

2 cups frozen corn

2 (4-ounce) cans chopped mild green chiles

3 cups low-sodium chicken broth or Slow Cooker Bone Broth (page 36)

1 cup whole milk

Meat from 1 whole chicken, cooked and chopped (about 3 cups)

2 cups shredded cheddar cheese

1. In a large stockpot, heat the oil over medium heat. Add the onion, celery, carrot, and mushrooms and sauté for about 5 minutes, or until softened. Stir in the garlic, cumin, paprika, salt, cayenne (if using), and black pepper and cook for another 1 to 2 minutes, or until fragrant.

2. Stir in the beans, corn, and chiles. Then add the broth and milk and stir to combine. Increase the heat to high and bring to a boil, then turn down the heat to low. Add the chicken and simmer for 10 minutes. Add the cheese, stir, and simmer for another 5 minutes.

3. Using a slotted spoon, scoop out 2 to 4 tablespoons of chicken and vegetables into a bowl, let cool, then serve to baby to eat with their hands or a spoon. Store leftovers in an airtight container in the refrigerator for up to 5 days or in the freezer for up to 5 months.

Sweet Potato Gnocchi with Browned Butter

NUT-FREE
SERVES: 4 | **PREP TIME:** 20 minutes | **COOK TIME:** 5 minutes

Gnocchi are fun, delicious potato pillows. We love them with brown butter and some sautéed vegetables (such as scallions and corn) or tossed with Simple Pesto (page 45) or tomato sauce. These sweet potato gnocchi are a twist on the traditional white potato version.

2 medium-large sweet potatoes, baked and cooled

1 large egg

½ teaspoon sea salt

1½ to 2 cups whole wheat flour or gluten-free flour, plus more for dusting

3 tablespoons unsalted butter

2 tablespoons Parmesan cheese

1. Fill a large stockpot three-quarters full of water and bring the water to a boil over medium-high heat.

2. Line a large baking sheet with parchment paper.

3. Scoop the baked sweet potato flesh into a large bowl and mash until smooth. Add the egg and salt, stirring thoroughly. Fold in the flour about ½ cup at a time, until a sticky but fairly cohesive dough has formed.

4. Liberally flour a clean work surface.

5. With floured hands, remove an egg-size chunk of the dough, rolling gently on the work surface to coat the exterior in flour. Roll the flour-covered dough into a long log, about ½ inch thick. Cut the dough with a sharp knife or pizza cutter into 1-inch sections. Put the raw gnocchi on the prepared baking sheet. Repeat this step with the remaining dough.

6. Put the gnocchi in the boiling water and cook them for 2 to 3 minutes, or until almost all the gnocchi float.

7. Meanwhile, make the sauce. In a small pan, melt the butter over medium heat. Stir frequently as the butter melts, then foams, then turns golden, and finally begins to brown and smell nutty. This should take about 5 minutes.

8. Toss the cooked gnocchi in the butter and sprinkle cheese over the top.

9. Allow 2 to 4 gnocchi to cool for baby, then cut them lengthwise and serve on a plate or tray to eat with their hands or a fork. Store leftovers in an airtight container in the refrigerator for up to 3 days.

TIP: Uncooked gnocchi can be frozen on the baking sheet and then transferred to an airtight container and frozen for up to 1 month. Cook when still frozen, adding about 1 minute to the boiling time.

Sloppy Joes with a Twist

DAIRY-FREE, GLUTEN-FREE, NUT-FREE
SERVES: 4+ | **PREP TIME:** 5 minutes | **COOK TIME:** 30 minutes

One of my favorite things to do is take "classic" dishes or comfort foods and find a way to make them a bit more nutritious. This recipe is a major palate-pleaser for my husband, and I'm a fan of the fiber. Try adding some leftover Chicken Liver Pâté (page 52) or mix in some minced chicken liver. Remember to check the label on your Worcestershire sauce; some brands contain soy sauce and, therefore, could contain gluten.

½ cup green lentils, rinsed and sorted

1 tablespoon avocado oil

½ sweet onion, finely diced

1 large carrot, finely diced

½ red bell pepper, finely diced

½ pound ground beef

¼ cup ketchup

2 tablespoons tomato paste

1 tablespoon gluten-free Worcestershire sauce

½ to 1 tablespoon maple syrup

1 teaspoon minced garlic

½ teaspoon ground mustard

Pinch sea salt

1. Cook the lentils according to the package instructions. (Typically, in a medium saucepan with 1 cup water over medium heat for 15 to 20 minutes, or until lentils are tender, but not mushy.) Drain.

2. Meanwhile, in a large skillet, heat the oil over medium heat. Add the onion and carrot and sauté for about 5 minutes, or until they begin to soften.

3. Add the bell pepper and ground beef. Cook, stirring and breaking up the meat, for about 5 minutes, or until the meat is browned. Turn down the heat to medium-low.

4. Add the ketchup, tomato paste, Worcestershire sauce, maple syrup, garlic, mustard, salt, and cooked lentils to the meat and vegetables. Simmer for 5 to 10 minutes, until it reaches your desired thickness. Taste and adjust the seasoning as desired.

5. Let 1 to 2 tablespoons cool, then serve it to baby on a plate or tray for them to eat with their hands or a spoon. Store leftovers in an airtight container in the refrigerator for up to 4 days or in the freezer for up to 6 months.

One-Pot Meatballs and Sauce

DAIRY-FREE, GLUTEN-FREE, NUT-FREE

SERVES: 4+ | **PREP TIME:** 10 minutes | **COOK TIME:** 30 minutes

I love one-pot meals. It makes cleanup so much easier, and after the prep, you can get back to doing whatever else needs to get done without being trapped in the kitchen. These meatballs are tender and flavorful; the sauce makes them a great texture for new eaters, too. Serve over macaroni for a baby-friendly twist on spaghetti and meatballs.

2 tablespoons avocado oil, divided

1 small yellow onion, finely diced

8 ounces mushrooms, stems removed and finely diced

1 small bell pepper, any color, seeded and finely diced

3 teaspoons minced garlic, divided

1 pound ground beef

3 ounces chicken liver, finely chopped

1 large egg

2 cups diced fresh spinach

1 teaspoon sea salt

½ teaspoon dried oregano

Pinch ground black pepper

1 (32-ounce) can crushed tomatoes or tomato puree

1. In a large stockpot, heat 1 tablespoon of the oil over medium heat. Add the onion, mushrooms, bell pepper, and 2 teaspoons of the garlic. Sauté for 5 minutes, or until lightly browned.

2. In a large bowl, combine the ground beef, liver, egg, spinach, salt, oregano, and black pepper. Add the cooked vegetables and mix well to combine.

3. In the same large stockpot, heat the remaining tablespoon of avocado oil over medium-high heat. Add the remaining teaspoon of garlic and cook, stirring, for 1 minute, or until fragrant. Turn down the heat to medium, add the crushed tomatoes, and allow to simmer while you form the meatballs.

4. Scoop 1 tablespoon of the meat mixture into your hands and form a meatball, then gently place each meatball into the tomato sauce. Repeat with the remaining meat mixture.

5. Cook at a low simmer, covered, for about 20 minutes, or until the meatballs are cooked through. Do not stir (stirring can cause the meatballs to fall apart).

6. Let 1 or 2 meatballs and sauce cool, then cut the meatballs into quarters and serve to baby on a plate or tray to eat with their hands, a fork, or a spoon. Store leftovers in an airtight container in the refrigerator for up to 4 days.

TIP: Make-ahead option: Place the uncooked meatballs on a parchment-paper-lined baking tray and freeze until solid. Transfer the meatballs to an airtight container and freeze for up to 4 months. To cook, add the meatballs to the sauce straight from the freezer and cook for 10 minutes longer, or until cooked through and the internal temperature reaches 165°F.

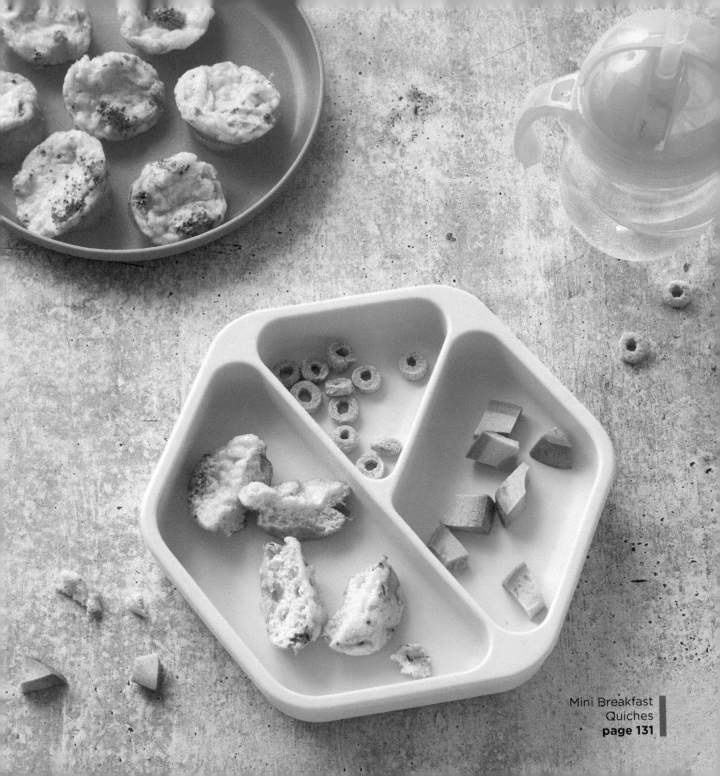

Mini Breakfast
Quiches
page 131

CHAPTER 6

Toddler Foods (12+ Months)

Avocado Seaweed Snacks

DAIRY-FREE, GLUTEN-FREE, NUT-FREE, VEGAN

SERVES: 4 | **PREP TIME:** 10 minutes

Seaweed is a great source of iodine, vitamins, and even a bit of iron. It has a crunch but dissolves fairly easily, making it a safe option for little eaters. Adding some avocado boosts the nutrition with more fiber, folate, and healthy fats. This is a great afternoon snack option, served alongside eggs for breakfast or grilled chicken and fruit for lunch.

1 (5-ounce) package dried seaweed

1 ripe avocado, pitted and thinly sliced

2 to 3 teaspoons everything bagel seasoning (optional)

2 teaspoons ground flaxseed (optional)

1. Cut each sheet of seaweed in half lengthwise. Top with 1 or 2 thin avocado slices. Repeat with the remaining strips of seaweed and avocado slices. Sprinkle desired toppings over the top, if using.

2. Serve baby 2 or 3 seaweed strips with avocado on a plate or tray to eat with their hands. Although you can safely store leftovers in an airtight container in the refrigerator for up to 2 days, the seaweed will get softer, and the avocado will start to brown.

TIP: We love gimMe and SeaSnax roasted seaweed snacks. Trader Joe's and Amazon both carry an "Everything Bagel" seasoning (that does contain sesame).

Homemade Granola Bars

DAIRY-FREE, GLUTEN-FREE

MAKES: 32 mini bars | **PREP TIME:** 15 minutes, plus 1 hour to chill

Granola bars are a simple snack to have on hand but are often full of added sugar—not these. I recommend adding collagen powder, as it drastically increases the protein. Note that these are *only* for little ones 12 months and older, because they include honey.

2 cups gluten-free oats

¼ to ⅓ cup honey

½ cup all-natural creamy peanut butter

¼ cup coconut oil, melted

2 to 4 tablespoons collagen powder (optional)

1 tablespoon ground flaxseed

1 tablespoon hemp seeds

½ cup mini chocolate chips

½ cup naturally dyed sprinkles (optional)

1. Line an 8-by-8-inch pan with parchment paper.

2. In a large bowl, mix all the ingredients together until well combined. The mixture should stick together well. If not, add a bit more peanut butter or coconut oil, and, if you'd like more sweetness, add more honey. Press the oat mixture into the prepared baking pan in an even layer. Chill for at least 1 hour. Cut into 2-by-1-inch bars.

3. Serve baby 1 bar at a time to eat with their hands. Store leftovers in an airtight container in the refrigerator for up to 5 days.

TIP: Straight out of the refrigerator, the bars can be a bit hard; just let them sit out for a few minutes to make them easier for baby to eat.

Avocado Toast Strips

DAIRY-FREE, NUT-FREE, VEGAN
SERVES: 4+ | **PREP TIME:** 15 minutes

Whether you serve it for breakfast, lunch, or dinner, avocado toast is a great base for a variety of toppings, such as fried eggs, smoked salmon, or turkey breast. For older eaters, you can top it with chopped kale, massaged with oil and lemon juice, or try arugula and thinly sliced radishes with a bit of oil and balsamic vinegar.

4 slices gluten-free or whole-grain bread

2 small ripe avocados, halved and pitted

½ teaspoon sea salt

¼ teaspoon ground black pepper

Juice of ½ lemon

Olive oil, for drizzling

1. Toast the bread to preferred crispness. Scoop half of an avocado onto each slice of toast and mash it with a fork until mostly smooth and spread evenly over the entire slice.

2. Season each piece with a bit of salt and pepper. Squeeze the lemon over each piece, then top with a drizzle of olive oil.

3. Cut a half or whole piece of toast into ½-inch strips and serve to baby to eat with their hands. This dish doesn't store well, so plan to eat it in one sitting, or halve the recipe if you plan for it to feed only yourself and baby.

Simple Slaw

DAIRY-FREE, GLUTEN-FREE, NUT-FREE, VEGAN

SERVES: 4+ | **PREP TIME:** 15 minutes, plus 30 minutes to chill

I love finding ways to get cruciferous vegetables into my kids' diets (and my own). This slaw comes together quickly with a shredding blade on a food processor. You can also shred it manually on the fine-shred side of a cheese grater, but it's *really* important that this be finely shredded (*not* the store-bought version) so it is appropriate for your little eater.

1 small head of cabbage, very finely shredded

2 scallions, white and green parts, finely sliced

3 tablespoons olive oil

2 tablespoons apple cider vinegar

Juice of ½ lime

Maple syrup, for drizzling

Pinch sea salt

Pinch ground black pepper

1. In a large bowl, combine the cabbage and scallions. Then add the oil, vinegar, lime juice, and a drizzle of maple syrup, then season with salt and pepper.

2. Toss with tongs or your hands until evenly mixed. Taste and adjust the flavors as desired. If you'd like it more acidic, add more vinegar or lime. For less acidic, add a bit more oil and salt or syrup.

3. Set aside in the refrigerator for at least 30 minutes to allow the flavors to meld.

4. Serve baby 2 tablespoons in a bowl to eat with their hands or a spoon. Store leftovers in an airtight container in the refrigerator for up to 3 days.

TIP: This is especially good with the Spiced Turkey Meatballs (page 140), the Banh Mi–Style Pulled Pork (page 143), or simple grilled chicken. If baby is struggling to scoop up the slaw, you can also mix it with a bit of mashed avocado to make it a bit "stickier" and easier to scoop.

Tomato Basil Salad

DAIRY-FREE, GLUTEN-FREE, NUT-FREE, VEGAN

SERVES: 4+ | **PREP TIME:** 15 minutes, plus 30 minutes to chill (optional)

Basil and tomatoes are one of the loveliest pairings of the summer. I do recommend chilling this salad to let the flavors meld, but it's not strictly required, and the dish is still delicious immediately after making. Try pairing this with some fresh mozzarella slices or feta cheese.

2 cups cherry tomatoes, quartered

1 to 2 tablespoons olive oil

1 to 2 tablespoons balsamic vinegar

1 teaspoon minced garlic

¼ cup fresh basil leaves, thinly sliced

Pinch sea salt

Pinch ground black pepper

1. In a small bowl, combine all the ingredients and toss gently. Taste and adjust the seasoning as desired. Chill for 30 minutes, if desired, before serving.

2. Serve baby 2 to 4 tablespoons on a plate or tray to eat with their hands or a spoon. Store leftovers in an airtight container in the refrigerator for up to 3 days.

Yogurt Bowls

GLUTEN-FREE, NUT-FREE, VEGETARIAN

SERVES: 4 | **PREP TIME:** 10 minutes

This is a breakfast staple in our house. It's simple to make, easy to adapt, and ensures everyone gets protein and healthy fats to start the day. For years, my kids called the chia seeds "sprinkles" and the bee pollen "yellow sprinkles." All the optional ingredients are delicious and have great health benefits, such as allergy support from the pollen and an immune boost from the elderberry syrup.

1 to 2 cups full-fat plain unsweetened yogurt

½ to 1 cup fresh or frozen berries, chopped if necessary (at least partially thawed if frozen)

2 to 3 tablespoons chia seeds

2 tablespoons hemp seeds

1 to 2 tablespoons ground flaxseed (optional)

1 tablespoon bee pollen (optional)

Maple syrup, for drizzling (optional)

Elderberry syrup, for drizzling (optional)

1. Spoon ¼ to ½ cup of yogurt into each of four bowls. Top each serving with equal portions of berries, chia seeds, and hemp seeds. Add the flaxseed, bee pollen, or a drizzle of maple syrup or elderberry syrup, if desired.

2. Serve baby ¼ cup (with toppings) in a bowl to eat with a spoon. Store leftovers in an airtight container in the refrigerator for up to 3 days.

ALLERGENS

Roasted Cauliflower with Lime

GLUTEN-FREE, NUT-FREE, VEGETARIAN

SERVES: 4+ | **PREP TIME:** 15 minutes | **COOK TIME:** 40 minutes

This cauliflower is rich, bright, and delicious. The brown butter really makes this dish; be sure to watch it closely, as it can go from perfect to burnt in a heartbeat.

1 large head of cauliflower, cut into ½-inch chunks (stem included)

2 tablespoons avocado oil

½ teaspoon sea salt

¼ teaspoon ground black pepper

3 tablespoons unsalted butter

Juice of ½ or 1 lime

1 scallion, white and green parts thinly sliced

1. Preheat the oven to 450°F. Line a baking sheet with parchment paper.

2. In a large bowl, toss the cauliflower with the oil, salt, and pepper, then pour it onto the prepared baking sheet and spread it in a single layer. Roast for 20 minutes, until the bottoms have started to brown well. Flip the pieces and roast for another 15 to 20 minutes, until tender and dark golden brown.

3. Meanwhile, make the sauce. In a small pan, melt the butter over medium heat, stirring as the butter melts, foams, and begins to brown and smell nutty, about 5 minutes.

4. When the cauliflower is roasted, season with the brown butter, lime juice, and scallion.

5. Let a few pieces of cauliflower cool and serve them to baby on a plate or tray to eat with their hands or a fork. Store leftovers in an airtight container in the refrigerator for up to 5 days.

Rice and Beans with Kimchi

DAIRY-FREE, GLUTEN-FREE, NUT-FREE, VEGAN

SERVES: 4 | **PREP TIME:** 15 minutes | **CHILL TIME:** 15 minutes

This has been a major kid-pleaser at our house. We use the Basic Cauliflower Rice but you can use regular rice or a mix of the two. Try it with a fried egg on top or some slices of fresh avocado.

2 tablespoons avocado oil

½ sweet onion, finely diced

1 teaspoon minced garlic

1 batch Basic Cauliflower Rice (page 97) or store-bought riced cauliflower

2 (15-ounce) cans no-salt-added kidney beans, pinto beans, black beans, or a mix, rinsed and drained

½ teaspoon ground cumin

¼ teaspoon sea salt

Pinch ground black pepper

2 to 4 tablespoons kimchi, finely diced

1. In a large skillet, heat the oil over medium heat. Add the onion and sauté, stirring occasionally, for about 5 minutes, or until it begins to soften and caramelize slightly.

2. Add the garlic and cook for another minute, or until the garlic is fragrant. Then add the cauliflower rice and cook for 5 to 8 minutes, or until heated through and the desired tenderness is reached.

3. Add the beans and cook, stirring, for about 2 minutes, or until the beans are warmed through. Stir in the cumin, salt, and pepper. Taste and adjust the seasoning as desired. Stir in the kimchi.

4. Let 2 to 4 tablespoons cool, then serve to baby on a plate or in a bowl to eat with their hands or a spoon. Store leftovers in an airtight container in the refrigerator for up to 4 days.

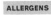

Cauliflower "Fried" Rice

DAIRY-FREE, GLUTEN-FREE, NUT-FREE, VEGETARIAN

SERVES: 4+ | **PREP TIME:** 10 minutes | **COOK TIME:** 15 minutes

Using cauliflower rice as the base for traditionally rice-based dishes is one of my favorite ways to increase fiber and vegetables in the diet. It also helps reduce heavy metals, because rice can be a pretty big arsenic risk. I recommend limiting it or doing half cauliflower rice and half regular rice. Add shrimp or chicken for a heartier, more protein-rich dish.

1 tablespoon avocado oil

½ sweet onion, diced

2 teaspoons minced garlic

2 teaspoons minced fresh ginger

½ bell pepper, any color, seeded and diced

1 carrot, shredded

½ cup peas, fresh or frozen

1 batch Basic Cauliflower Rice (page 97) or store-bought riced cauliflower

2 tablespoons gluten-free tamari

1 teaspoon apple cider vinegar or white vinegar

2 teaspoons toasted sesame oil

2 large eggs, lightly beaten

1. In a large skillet, heat the avocado oil over medium-high heat. Add the onion, garlic, and ginger. Cook, stirring, for 1 minute, or until fragrant.

2. Turn down the heat to medium and add the bell pepper, carrot, and peas. Cook for about 3 minutes, or until the vegetables begin to soften.

3. If using uncooked cauliflower rice, add it now. Stir in the tamari and vinegar. Cook for another 3 minutes, until the cauliflower is softening.

4. Make a well in the middle of the vegetables and add the sesame oil. Increase the heat to medium-high and pour the eggs into the well. Scramble the eggs, gradually mixing them into the vegetable mix. If using already-cooked cauliflower rice, add it now and cook until everything is heated through.

5. Let 2 to 4 tablespoons cool, then serve to baby on a plate or in a bowl to eat with their hands or a spoon. Store leftovers in an airtight container in the refrigerator for up to 4 days.

Crustless Asparagus Bacon Quiche

GLUTEN-FREE, NUT-FREE
SERVES: 4+ | **PREP TIME:** 15 minutes | **COOK TIME:** 1 hour

Quiche is a great way to incorporate vegetables. Try sautéed leeks and sausage or roasted red peppers with caramelized onion. This recipe is very adaptable—a great way to use whatever you've got in your refrigerator.

8 to 10 ounces bacon, diced

8 large eggs

1 cup whole milk

1 cup very thinly sliced asparagus, bottoms trimmed

2 cups shredded cheddar cheese

¼ teaspoon sea salt

Pinch ground black pepper

1. Preheat the oven to 375°F. Lightly grease an 8-by-8-inch or 9-inch cake pan.

2. In a large skillet over medium-low heat, cook the bacon for 10 to 15 minutes, stirring periodically, until crisp.

3. Meanwhile, in a large bowl, whisk together the eggs and milk until thoroughly combined. Stir in the asparagus, cheese, salt, and pepper.

4. When the bacon is crisped, use a slotted spoon to scoop it from the pan, add it to the egg mixture, and stir. Pour the egg mixture into the prepared pan. Bake for 35 to 40 minutes, or until the eggs are set. Let cool for at least 5 minutes before serving.

5. Serve baby a 2-by-1-inch piece of quiche on a plate or tray to eat with their hands or a fork. Store leftovers in an airtight container in the refrigerator for up to 4 days.

Mini Breakfast Quiches

GLUTEN-FREE, NUT-FREE

MAKES: 16 to 18 regular muffins or 30 mini muffins | **PREP TIME:** 10 minutes | **COOK TIME:** 25 minutes

I love these for a quick, simple breakfast that's both filling and full of protein and vegetables. Because it's in muffin form, many little ones are super happy to try it. It's a great option to grab when you're on the run or to pack for lunch.

Avocado oil, for greasing

12 large eggs

¾ cup whole milk

1½ cups shredded sharp cheddar cheese

1 cup diced fresh or frozen broccoli (thawed and drained if frozen)

2 tablespoons finely diced chives

¼ teaspoon sea salt

Pinch ground black pepper

1. Preheat the oven to 375°F. Grease a muffin tin (regular or mini) liberally with avocado oil. In a large bowl, whisk together the eggs and milk. Stir in the cheese, broccoli, chives, salt, and pepper.

2. Fill the muffin cups three-quarters full. Bake for 15 to 20 minutes for mini quiches or 20 to 25 minutes for regular muffins, or until the egg is set and the quiches are beginning to brown on the top. Let cool in the pan for 5 minutes. Gently run a butter knife around each muffin and transfer them to a cooling rack to cool completely.

3. Serve baby large muffins cut into strips or mini muffins cut into halves or quarters on a plate to eat with their hands. Store leftovers in an airtight container in the refrigerator for up to 4 days. To freeze, arrange the cooled quiches on a sheet pan and freeze. Once frozen, transfer them to an airtight container and freeze for up to 3 months.

Fish Sticks

DAIRY-FREE, GLUTEN-FREE

SERVES: 4+ | **PREP TIME:** 15 minutes | **COOK TIME:** 20 minutes

Fish sticks are a kid favorite. This version is simple to make, tastes awesome, is naturally gluten-free, and uses brain-building omega-3-rich fish. The tartar sauce is great for dipping, plus it offers a probiotic boost. For a complete meal, serve these with the Simple Slaw (page 123).

For the fish

Avocado oil cooking spray

2 large eggs

1 teaspoon gluten-free tamari

¾ teaspoon sea salt, divided

½ teaspoon ground black pepper, divided

1½ cups almond flour

3 tablespoons tapioca flour

½ teaspoon paprika

½ teaspoon onion powder

1 pound cod, fresh or frozen (thawed), cut into 2-inch-by-½-inch strips

For the tartar sauce

¾ cup mayonnaise

¼ heaping cup dill sauerkraut, finely chopped

3 tablespoons diced sweet onion

1 tablespoon capers, chopped

1 teaspoon maple syrup

Pinch ground black pepper

TO MAKE THE FISH

1. Preheat the oven to 425°F. Line a large baking sheet with parchment paper. Spray the paper with a thin layer of avocado oil.

2. In a medium bowl, whisk the eggs with tamari, half the salt, and half the pepper.

3. In a small shallow bowl or pan, mix together the almond flour, tapioca flour, paprika, onion powder, and the remaining salt and pepper.

4. Dip a strip of the cod into the egg mixture, allow excess to drip off, coat it with the almond flour mixture, and place it on the prepared baking sheet. Continue with the remaining fish strips, leaving an inch or two between each strip.

5. Spray the top of the fish sticks lightly with more avocado oil, then bake for 8 minutes. Flip and bake for another 6 to 8 minutes, or until the fish is flaky and the coating is starting to brown.

TO MAKE THE TARTAR SAUCE

6. While the fish sticks bake, in a small bowl, mix together all the tartar sauce ingredients.

TO SERVE

7. Allow 1 or 2 fish sticks to cool, then serve to baby as is or cut into bite-size pieces, along with a tablespoon of tartar sauce to eat with their hands. Store leftovers in an airtight container in the refrigerator for up to 2 days. Reheat before serving.

Canned Salmon Salad

GLUTEN-FREE, NUT-FREE

SERVES: 4+ | **PREP TIME:** 15 minutes

Tuna salad is well-known, but why not salmon salad? Salmon is rich in healthy, anti-inflammatory, brain-boosting fats and is a great source of protein. Unlike tuna, there are no concerns about "overdoing" it because of mercury content. We love this on almond flour crackers like SimpleMills, on cucumber or apple slice rounds (for adults and older eaters), or on top of a bed of mixed greens.

15 ounces canned, no-salt-added salmon

¼ heaping cup full-fat plain unsweetened yogurt or sour cream

1 to 2 tablespoons everything bagel seasoning

1 tablespoon capers, chopped

¼ teaspoon ground black pepper

1. In a medium bowl, mix together all the ingredients until well combined. Taste and adjust the seasoning as desired.

2. Serve baby 2 to 4 tablespoons on a plate or tray to eat with their hands or a spoon. Store leftovers in an airtight container in the refrigerator for up to 4 days.

Simple Chicken Salad

DAIRY-FREE, GLUTEN-FREE, NUT-FREE

SERVES: 4+ | **PREP TIME:** 10 minutes | **COOK TIME:** 15 minutes

Serve this chicken salad as is for new eaters and, for older family members, on croissants, crackers, or a bed of greens. No mixer? Let the chicken cool until it's easy to handle, then use two forks to finely shred the chicken breast.

2 pounds chicken breast, each breast halved

½ cup green grapes, finely diced

1 celery stalk, finely diced

2 scallions, white and green parts, finely sliced

¾ to 1 cup mayonnaise

2 teaspoons Dijon mustard

½ teaspoon sea salt

¼ to ½ teaspoon ground black pepper

1. Fill a large pot halfway full of water and bring it to a boil over high heat. Slip the chicken breasts into the boiling water, and boil them for 10 to 15 minutes, or until the chicken reaches an internal temperature of 165°F.

2. Drain the chicken and put it into the bowl of a stand mixer. Cover the mixer with a towel to help contain the steam and the chicken. Starting on low speed, use the mixer to shred the chicken. Increase the speed slightly and continue mixing and shredding for about 3 minutes, or until the chicken is very finely shredded.

3. Turn down the speed to low and add the grapes, celery, scallions, mayonnaise, mustard, salt, and pepper. Mix until well combined.

4. Serve baby 2 to 4 tablespoons on a plate or tray to eat with their hands or a fork. Store leftovers in an airtight container in the refrigerator for up to 4 days.

Sweet Potato Nachos

GLUTEN-FREE, NUT-FREE, VEGETARIAN

SERVES: 4+ | **PREP TIME:** 15 minutes | **COOK TIME:** 35 minutes

Nachos are a delicious, fun family dinner, but they're not very baby-friendly with crunchy, hard chips. This recipe takes some of the best elements of nachos, increases the nutrition, and removes the choking hazards (chips). Add your favorite proteins (ground beef, shredded chicken, pork, even shrimp), cheeses, vegetables (pickled onions, bell peppers, Brussels sprouts), or whatever your go-to nacho fixings might be.

4 medium sweet potatoes (about 2 pounds), cut into ¼-inch slices

2 to 3 tablespoons avocado oil

½ to 1 teaspoon ground cumin

¼ to ½ teaspoon sea salt

1 (15-ounce) can no-salt-added black or pinto beans

2 cups shredded cheddar or Colby Jack cheese

1 cup cherry tomatoes, thinly sliced or quartered

1 ripe avocado, pitted and cubed

3 scallions, white and green parts, thinly sliced

¼ cup fresh cilantro leaves, coarsely torn

¼ to ½ cup sour cream or plain unsweetened full-fat yogurt (optional)

1. Preheat the oven to 400°F. Line a large baking sheet with parchment paper.

2. In a large bowl, toss the sweet potato slices with the oil, cumin, and salt. Spread evenly on the prepared baking sheet.

3. Roast the sweet potatoes for 15 minutes, until they begin to brown on the bottom, then flip and roast for another 10 to 15 minutes, or until tender.

4. Top with the beans and cheese. Bake for another 5 minutes, or until the cheese has melted and is bubbly. Remove from the oven and top with the tomatoes, avocado, scallions, cilantro, and sour cream.

5. Coarsely chop a few slices of loaded potatoes and let cool, then serve to baby on a plate or tray to eat with their hands or a fork. Store leftovers in an airtight container in the refrigerator for up to 4 days.

Egg Roll–Inspired Bowls

DAIRY-FREE, GLUTEN-FREE, NUT-FREE
SERVES: 4+ | **PREP TIME:** 15 minutes | **COOK TIME:** 20 minutes

Vegetable-packed, this recipe can be prepared with a knife or cheese grater, but a food processor greatly simplifies and speeds up the process. It's also a great way to incorporate vegetables such as cabbage and kale that can be hard to get kids to eat.

1 small or ½ large napa or
  green cabbage

1 bunch kale, center stems removed

4 ounces mushrooms, stems removed

3 or 4 medium carrots

3 tablespoons gluten-free tamari, divided

2 tablespoons avocado oil

1 pound ground pork

1 sweet onion, finely diced

2 teaspoons minced garlic

1 teaspoon peeled, finely diced
  fresh ginger

3 or 4 scallions, white and green parts,
  thinly sliced

2 to 3 teaspoons toasted sesame oil

2 teaspoons mirin or rice vinegar

1 teaspoon apple cider vinegar

1. Cut the cabbage, kale, mushrooms, and carrots into thin slices or run them through a food processor with the shredding disk until everything is evenly shredded.

2. In a large stockpot over medium heat, combine 2 tablespoons of the tamari with the avocado oil and then add the ground pork. Cook for 5 to 7 minutes, stirring and breaking up the meat, until it is browned.

3. Add the onion, garlic, and ginger. Cook for 2 to 3 minutes, or until fragrant. Then add the cabbage, kale, carrots, and mushrooms. Add the scallions, the remaining 1 tablespoon tamari, the sesame oil, the mirin, and the apple cider vinegar. Cook, stirring periodically for about 5 minutes, or until the greens are wilted but still have a slight crunch.

4. Let 1 to 2 tablespoons cool, then serve to baby on a plate or tray to eat with their hands or a spoon. Store leftovers in an airtight container in the refrigerator for up to 5 days.

TIP: You can change up the protein using tofu for a vegan option.

Spiced Turkey Meatballs

GLUTEN-FREE, NUT-FREE

SERVES: 4 | **PREP TIME:** 10 minutes | **COOK TIME:** 20 minutes

The meatballs have a touch of heat, so if you're concerned about the spice level, I recommend using just a pinch of cayenne. For the oats, a quick pulse in the food processor, blender, or spice grinder will do the trick.

1 pound ground turkey

⅓ cup coarsely ground gluten-free oats

⅓ cup ground flaxseed

¼ cup full-fat plain unsweetened yogurt

Pinch sea salt

1 large egg

2 teaspoons minced garlic

½ teaspoon ground cumin

½ teaspoon ground coriander

½ teaspoon paprika

¼ to ½ teaspoon cayenne

2 tablespoons toasted sesame seeds

1. Preheat the oven to 400°F. Line a baking sheet with parchment paper.

2. Put all the ingredients into a medium bowl and mix until well combined. Roll the meatballs into golf ball–size balls and place them 1 inch or so apart on the prepared baking sheet. Bake until cooked through and starting to brown, 12 to 15 minutes.

3. Let 1 or 2 meatballs cool, then cut them into quarters and serve to baby on a plate or tray to eat with their hands or a fork. Store leftovers in an airtight container in the refrigerator for up to 4 days.

TIP: Before baking, you can freeze the meatballs on the pan, then transfer to an airtight container to freeze for up to 3 months. Cook from frozen, adding about 5 minutes to the cook time. The meatballs are done when the internal temperature reaches 165°F.

Lamb Oven Meatballs

DAIRY-FREE, GLUTEN-FREE, NUT-FREE

SERVES: 4+ | **PREP TIME:** 10 minutes | **COOK TIME:** 15 minutes

Meatballs are a great protein option for new eaters, thanks to their soft texture. I'm a big fan of introducing kids to a wide variety of flavors, foods, and textures from the beginning, and you can absolutely substitute grass-fed ground beef or venison instead.

1 pound ground lamb

1 large egg

½ small sweet onion, finely diced

Juice and zest of ½ lemon

1 tablespoon dried parsley

2 heaping teaspoons garlic

1 heaping teaspoon ground cumin

⅛ to ¼ teaspoon ground black pepper

Pinch sea salt

1. Preheat the oven to 400°F. Line a baking sheet with parchment paper.

2. In a medium bowl, combine all the ingredients. Mix thoroughly, then scoop 1 tablespoon of meatball mixture into your hands and roll it into a ball. Place it on the prepared baking sheet. Repeat this step with the remaining meat mixture, spacing the meatballs about 1 inch apart.

3. Bake for 10 to 15 minutes, or until cooked through and the internal temperature reaches 165°F.

4. Let one or two meatballs cool, then cut them into quarters and serve to baby on a plate or tray to eat with their hands or a fork. Store leftovers in an airtight container in the refrigerator for up to 4 days. To reheat, see the tip on page 140.

Thai-Inspired Basil Beef

DAIRY-FREE, GLUTEN-FREE, NUT-FREE

SERVES: 4+ | **PREP TIME:** 5 minutes | **COOK TIME:** 15 minutes

Iron-rich and full of flavor for little ones and caregivers alike, this dish is also great with ground pork or lamb, if you want to switch it up. I also love that you get a huge helping of spinach and won't even notice it.

3 to 4 tablespoons avocado oil, divided

1 jalapeño pepper, seeds removed, minced

1 heaping tablespoon minced garlic

Pinch sea salt

1 pound ground beef

1 (5-ounce) bag fresh spinach, coarsely chopped

2 to 3 cups fresh basil leaves, very loosely packed, coarsely chopped

2 tablespoons fish sauce

Maple syrup, for drizzling

⅓ cup Slow Cooker Bone Broth (page 36), store-bought broth, or water

Juice of 1 lime

1. In a large skillet, heat 2 tablespoons of avocado oil over high heat. Add the jalapeño, garlic, and salt and sauté for 1 minute, or until fragrant.

2. Add the beef and cook for about 5 minutes, stirring and breaking up the meat, until the meat is browned. Add the spinach, basil, fish sauce, and a drizzle of maple syrup. Top with the broth. Stir until the greens are just wilted, about 2 minutes. Squeeze lime juice over the top.

3. Let 2 to 4 tablespoons cool, then serve to baby on a plate or tray to eat with their hands or a spoon. Store leftovers in an airtight container in the refrigerator for up to 4 days.

TIP: Serve over Basic Cauliflower Rice (page 97) or store-bought riced cauliflower, with a fried egg.

Banh Mi–Style Pulled Pork

DAIRY-FREE, GLUTEN-FREE, NUT-FREE
SERVES: 4+ | **PREP TIME:** 5 minutes | **COOK TIME:** 5 to 7 hours

Slow-cooked meat is a great for new eaters. It's a hands-off meal-prep option that produces a ton of flavor. No slow cooker? Cook, covered, in a 325°F oven for 2 to 3 hours until tender and falling apart.

2 pounds boneless pork shoulder

½ teaspoon sea salt

¼ teaspoon ground black pepper

1 small sweet onion, thinly sliced

2 heaping tablespoons minced garlic

2 tablespoons peeled and minced fresh ginger

⅓ cup maple syrup

4 tablespoons gluten-free tamari

4 tablespoons white vinegar or apple cider vinegar

2 tablespoons fish sauce

1. Season the pork with salt and pepper. Place the onion, garlic, ginger, maple syrup, tamari, vinegar, and fish sauce into a slow cooker. Place the pork on top.

2. Cover and cook on high for 1 to 2 hours, or until the liquid is bubbling. Turn down the heat to low and cook for another 4 to 5 hours, or until the pork is tender and falling apart.

3. Move the pork to a cutting board and shred, discarding any large chunks of fat. Strain the remaining cooking liquid into a bowl to use as a sauce.

4. Chop pork into 1-inch pieces. Let 2 tablespoons cool, then serve to baby on a plate or tray for them to eat with their hands or a fork. Store leftovers in an airtight container in the refrigerator for up to 4 days.

TIP: Serve with Simple Slaw (see page 123) or a mix of fresh vegetables (cucumber, carrots, or lettuce for wraps) for adults and older eaters.

Sheet Pan Meat Loaf and Roasted Veggies

DAIRY-FREE, GLUTEN-FREE, NUT-FREE

SERVES: 4+ | **PREP TIME:** 15 minutes | **COOK TIME:** 1 hour

Meat loaf is one of those comforting dishes that is perfect for a cold evening dinner. This version, with the vegetables and main roasting together, makes it easy to get a meal on the table without spending hours working over the stove. Then you can finish working, check some emails, or just cozy up with your kiddo for another reading of *Go, Dog. Go!*

2 pounds vegetables, cut into bite-size pieces (carrots, cabbage, Brussels sprouts, broccoli)

2 tablespoons avocado oil

½ teaspoon sea salt, divided

¼ teaspoon ground black pepper

8 ounces ground beef

2 to 3 ounces chicken liver, minced (optional)

1 large egg

1 small sweet onion, finely diced

1 small red bell pepper, finely diced

4 ounces mushrooms, finely diced

½ cup gluten-free oats

2 tablespoons ground flaxseed

1 teaspoon thyme

½ cup ketchup, divided

1. Preheat the oven to 375°F. Line a baking sheet with parchment paper.

2. In a large bowl, mix together the vegetables, oil, ¼ teaspoon of salt, and the pepper. Transfer to the prepared baking sheet, leaving an 8-inch-by-4-inch space in the center of the pan for the meat loaf.

3. In the same large bowl, combine the beef, liver (if using), egg, onion, bell pepper, mushrooms, oats, flaxseed, and thyme. Mix well.

4. Using your hands, form the meat mixture into an 8-inch-by-4-inch log, about 2 inches high, in the center of the prepared baking sheet. Coat the outside of the loaf with half the ketchup.

5. Bake for 40 minutes, then flip the vegetables and coat the meat loaf with the remaining ketchup. Bake for another 15 to 20 minutes, or until the internal temperature of the meat loaf reaches 165°F and the vegetables are golden brown.

6. Let a ½-inch-thick slice of meat loaf and 2 tablespoons of vegetables cool. Cut the meat into bite-size chunks or strips and serve to baby on a plate or tray to eat with their hands or a fork. Store leftovers in an airtight container in the refrigerator for up to 4 days.

Chocolate PB Avocado Pudding

DAIRY-FREE, GLUTEN-FREE, VEGAN

MAKES: About 1 cup | **PREP TIME:** 10 minutes, plus 30 minutes to chill

Chocolate pudding is a childhood staple, but it tends to be laden with sugar, corn syrup, and even food dyes. This is a superb alternative that both adults and kids will love full of healthy fats, fiber, and just a touch of natural sweetener. No food processor? Mash the avocado until smooth with a fork, then whisk in the remaining ingredients until smooth.

1 ripe avocado, pitted and halved

2 tablespoons maple syrup or Date Paste (page 40)

1 tablespoon all-natural creamy peanut butter

1 heaping tablespoon coconut oil

2 teaspoons hemp seeds

2 tablespoons cocoa powder

½ teaspoon vanilla extract

½ teaspoon ground flaxseed

¼ cup nut milk of choice (optional)

1. Put the avocado flesh into a food processor. Add the maple syrup, peanut butter, coconut oil, and hemp seeds. Process until very smooth, about 2 minutes. Scrape down the sides as needed.

2. Add the cocoa powder, vanilla, and flaxseed. Process again until very smooth and fluffy, another 2 to 3 minutes, stopping to scrape the sides periodically with a spatula. If you'd like a thinner consistency, drizzle in the milk a bit at a time while processing to reach your desired thickness. Spoon the pudding into an airtight container and set aside in the refrigerator to chill for at least 30 minutes.

3. Once chilled, serve baby 2 to 4 tablespoons in a bowl with a spoon. Store leftovers in an airtight container in the refrigerator for up to 4 days.

Anytime Cookies

DAIRY-FREE, GLUTEN-FREE

MAKES: About 12 cookies | **PREP TIME:** 10 minutes | **COOK TIME:** 15 minutes

These cookies are a win-win. Your kiddos feel as though they're getting a special treat, and *you* know they're actually getting healthy fats, fiber, and more. Snack, dessert, or even breakfast—these cookies are perfect.

1½ cups walnuts

1 cup Medjool dates, pitted (about 12)

¼ teaspoon sea salt

1 teaspoon vanilla extract

1 tablespoon ground flaxseed

4 tablespoons water

1 tablespoon collagen powder (optional)

½ cup gluten-free oats

2 tablespoons hemp seeds

¼ cup diced dried apricots or cherries

½ cup dairy-free dark chocolate chips

1. Preheat the oven to 350°F. Line a baking sheet with parchment paper.

2. Put the walnuts and dates in a food processor and process until crumbly. Add the salt, vanilla, flaxseed, water, and collagen, then process again until a smooth dough begins to form. Add the oats, hemp seeds, and apricots. Pulse until well mixed. Finally add the chocolate chips, pulsing briefly to distribute the chips.

3. Spoon heaping tablespoons of the batter onto the lined sheets. Wet your hands slightly to prevent sticking, then gently flatten the cookies.

4. Bake for 10 to 12 minutes, or until the edges are starting to turn golden brown. Allow to cool completely on the pan.

5. Serve baby one cookie to eat with their hands. Store leftovers in an airtight container in the refrigerator for up to 4 days.

Flourless Chocolate Cake

GLUTEN-FREE, NUT-FREE, VEGETARIAN

MAKES: 1 (6-inch) round cake | **PREP TIME:** 15 minutes | **COOK TIME:** 35 minutes

This was our son's second birthday cake. If you're looking for a light and fluffy cake, this is not your cake. It's rich, fudgy, and dense. If you're looking for a decadent and moist cake, this is it.

Oil or butter, for greasing

4 tablespoons unsalted butter

3 ounces semisweet chocolate, finely chopped

⅓ cup Date Paste (page 40)

2 large eggs

1 teaspoon vanilla extract

2 heaping tablespoons cocoa powder

¼ teaspoon ground cinnamon

Pinch sea salt

1. Preheat the oven to 350°F. Line the bottom of a 6-inch cake pan with parchment paper, then butter or oil the parchment paper and sides of the pan.

2. Cut the butter into pieces and put the pieces into a small microwave-safe bowl. Add the chocolate and microwave in 30-second increments, stirring after each, until the chocolate and butter are completely melted and smooth. Let cool for 3 minutes.

3. Meanwhile, in a large bowl, whisk together the date paste, eggs, and vanilla until smooth and a bit fluffy, 1 to 2 minutes. Pour in the slightly cooled chocolate mixture and whisk until smooth. The batter will be thick.

4. Add the cocoa powder, cinnamon, and salt and whisk again until fully combined. Pour the batter into the prepared dish and spread it in an even layer.

5. Bake for about 30 minutes, checking in around the 25-minute mark, until the edges are set and a toothpick inserted into the center comes out mostly clean (a few crumbs are okay).

6. Cool for 10 minutes in the pan, then run a butter knife around the edges to release the cake and invert it onto the serving plate. Let the cake cool completely before serving.

7. Serve a small slice to baby on a plate or tray to eat with their hands or a fork. Store leftovers in an airtight container in the refrigerator for up to 4 days.

TIP: This cake is perfection as is, but adding some Dairy-Free Whipped Cream (page 59) or store-bought whipped cream wouldn't hurt. Try it with fresh berries for a bit of tanginess to cut through the richness.

Sweet Potato Birthday Cake

DAIRY-FREE, GLUTEN-FREE, VEGETARIAN

MAKES: 2 (6-inch) round cakes | **PREP TIME:** 10 minutes | **COOK TIME:** 40 minutes

I am all for celebrating birthdays, and celebrating *big*, but your little one doesn't yet know that super-sugary, over-the-top cakes exist. They will absolutely adore this sweet but still nourishing option. To cook the sweet potato quickly, pierce it 3 or 4 times with a fork and microwave it for 5 to 8 minutes, until tender throughout.

2 tablespoons avocado oil, plus more for greasing

¾ cup cooked and peeled sweet potatoes (about 1 medium sweet potato)

½ cup Date Paste (page 40)

1 cup almond flour

½ cup arrowroot flour or cornstarch

3 large eggs

¼ cup all-natural creamy almond butter

2 teaspoons vanilla extract

1½ teaspoons baking soda

1½ teaspoons baking powder

1½ teaspoons ground cinnamon

¼ teaspoon ground nutmeg

¼ teaspoon ground ginger

Dash ground cardamom

Pinch sea salt

1. Preheat the oven to 350°F. Line the bottom of two 6-inch round pans with parchment paper and grease the paper and sides of the pan lightly with avocado oil.

2. Combine all the ingredients in a food processor or blender. Process until smooth and fluffy, 2 to 3 minutes, scraping down the sides as needed.

3. Spread half the batter into one prepared pan; repeat with the other half in the second pan. Bake for 30 or 40 minutes, or until the tops are golden and a toothpick inserted in the center comes out clean. Let cool for 10 minutes in the pan on cooling rack, then invert the cake onto the rack to cool completely.

4. Once cool, place one layer of the cake on a serving plate and frost as desired. Top with the second layer and then frost the exterior of both layers.

5. Serve baby a slice on a plate or tray to eat with their hands or a fork. Store leftovers in an airtight container in the refrigerator for up to 4 days.

TIP: You can use a conventional frosting with this, but I recommend something a bit lighter, like Dairy-Free Whipped Cream (page 59) or the Avocado Chocolate Frosting (page 153).

Banana Cake

DAIRY-FREE, GLUTEN-FREE, VEGETARIAN

MAKES: 1 (9-by-13-inch) cake | **PREP TIME:** 10 minutes | **COOK TIME:** 35 minutes

No 12-month chapter would be complete without some recipes for the big first birthday. You can top this cake with the chocolate whipped cream or Avocado Chocolate Frosting (page 153). No mixer? Mash the bananas very smooth and warm the almond butter until drippy; then stir everything together until well combined.

3 very ripe bananas, mashed

3 large eggs

1 cup all-natural creamy almond butter

½ teaspoon baking soda

½ teaspoon ground cinnamon

Pinch sea salt

1. Preheat the oven to 350°F. Line a 9-by-13-inch pan with parchment paper.

2. In the bowl of a stand mixer, mix the banana with the eggs for about 3 minutes, or until smooth and fluffy. Add the almond butter, baking soda, cinnamon, and salt and mix again until smooth and thoroughly combined, another 2 to 3 minutes. Pour the batter into the prepared dish and spread it in an even layer.

3. Bake for 30 to 35 minutes, or until the top has browned and the center is set. Allow the cake to cool completely in the pan, then lift the cake out of the pan using the parchment paper. Frost as desired.

4. Serve baby a small square of the cake on a plate or tray to eat with their hands or a fork. Store leftovers in an airtight container in the refrigerator for up to 4 days.

TIP: Add mini chocolate chips for a fun chocolate twist, or try peanut butter in place of the almond butter for a peanut butter option.

Avocado Chocolate Frosting

DAIRY-FREE, GLUTEN-FREE, VEGAN

MAKES: About 2 cups | **PREP TIME:** 10 minutes, plus 15 minutes to chill

We love this spread on the Sweet Potato Birthday Cake (page 150) and use it to make regular muffins a bit more "fancy" (such as the Double Chocolate Chip Veggie Muffins, page 90). No food processor? This can be made in a mixer if you use a *very* ripe avocado and chop it up first.

2 ripe avocados, halved and pitted

¾ cup cocoa powder

⅓ cup maple syrup, plus more as needed

2 tablespoons coconut oil, melted

Pinch sea salt

1. Put the avocado flesh in a food processor and process until smooth. Scrape down the sides of the food processor and add the cocoa powder, maple syrup, coconut oil, and salt. Process until the frosting is very smooth and starts to get glossy, about 3 minutes. Stop and scrape down the sides as needed.

2. Taste and adjust the sweetness, as desired, and reprocess if needed. Set aside in the refrigerator to chill for 15 minutes, if needed, to reach desired spreading or piping consistency.

3. Serve baby 1 or 2 tablespoons in a bowl to eat with a spoon, or use it to frost your desired treat. Store leftovers in an airtight container in the refrigerator for up to 3 days.

TIP: Try adding all-natural creamy peanut butter for a chocolate-peanut butter twist or even a pinch of cinnamon and paprika for a Mexican chocolate-inspired option.

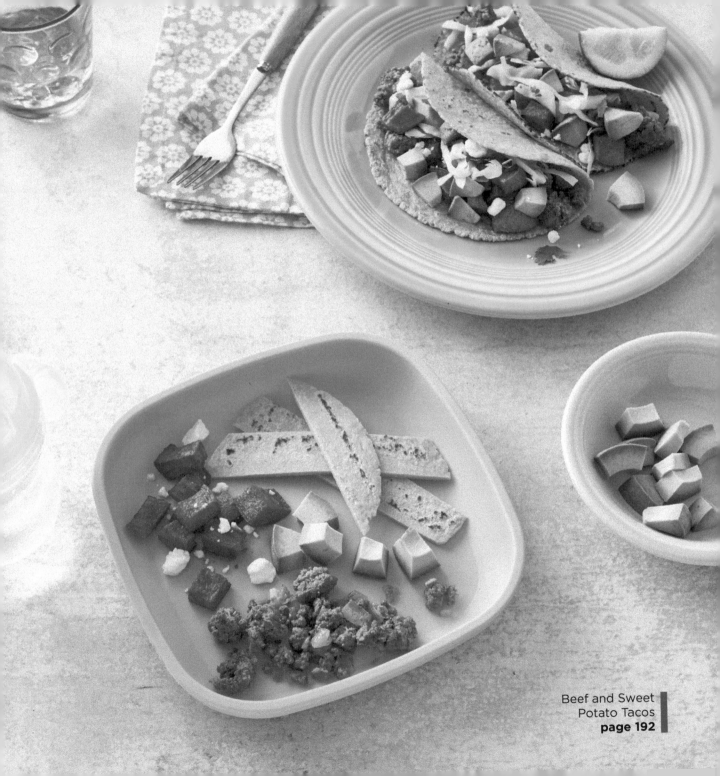

Beef and Sweet
Potato Tacos
page 192

CHAPTER 7

At the Family Table (15+ Months)

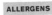

Chocolate PB Banana Smoothie Bowl

GLUTEN-FREE

MAKES: 2 bowls | **PREP TIME:** 10 minutes

Smoothie bowls are one of my go-to options when I don't want to cook and need to get something other than cereal on the table ASAP. My kids think they're a fun treat, and I love that they're packed with all sorts of good-for-you ingredients.

2 ripe bananas, chopped into large chunks

2 giant handfuls fresh or frozen spinach

½ cup full-fat plain unsweetened yogurt

2 heaping tablespoons cocoa powder

2 tablespoons collagen powder (optional)

½ teaspoon ground cinnamon

½ to 1 cup whole milk

4 to 6 ice cubes

Optional toppings

All-natural creamy peanut butter, melted

Chia seeds

Hemp seeds

Fresh berry pieces

Mini chocolate chips

Cacao nibs

Chopped unsalted peanuts

Dairy-Free Whipped Cream (page 59) or store-bought whipped cream

1. Put the bananas, spinach, yogurt, cocoa powder, collagen (if using), and cinnamon into a blender. Starting on the lowest speed, begin to blend, using the tamper to push things down.

2. Drizzle in the milk, a tiny bit at a time, just to keep the blender moving. If you use too much, you'll get a smoothie instead of a smoothie bowl, so go slow. Continue blending, adding liquid slowly as needed until smooth. Add the ice and blend again until smooth and frosty.

3. Serve baby 2 to 4 tablespoons in a bowl to start, topped with baby-friendly toppings of choice to eat with their spoon. Leftovers can be poured into ice pop molds and frozen for up to a month.

TIP: Did you add too much liquid? Add a tablespoon or two of peanut butter, chia seeds, and hemp seeds, if desired, and blend again for a drinkable smoothie.

Quinoa Cakes

NUT-FREE

MAKES: About 12 cakes | **PREP TIME:** 10 minutes | **COOK TIME:** 15 minutes

Quinoa is a protein and fiber-rich seed, often used like a grain. These cakes are a kid-friendly way to serve quinoa, as it tends to be messy and difficult for newer eaters to manage. The quinoa and spinach offer an iron boost, especially with the vitamin C from the lemon helping increase absorption.

2 cups cooked quinoa

1 cup fresh spinach, finely chopped

3 large eggs

½ cup panko bread crumbs

¼ cup shredded Parmesan cheese (optional)

1 tablespoon dried parsley

1 tablespoon ground flaxseed

Juice and zest of 1 lemon

2 teaspoons minced garlic

½ teaspoon sea salt

¼ teaspoon ground black pepper

1. Preheat the oven to 375°F. Line a baking sheet with parchment paper.

2. In a large bowl, mix together all the ingredients until thoroughly combined. Scoop 2 tablespoons of quinoa mixture into your hands and form it into a patty. Place the patty on the prepared sheet. Repeat with the remaining quinoa mix, leaving about 1 inch between patties.

3. Bake for 10 minutes, then broil for about 3, until the tops are golden. Let cool until easy to handle.

4. Serve baby one patty, cut into strips or bite-size pieces, on a plate or tray to eat with their hands or fork. Store leftovers in an airtight container in the refrigerator for up to 5 days.

TIP: These are great with a fried egg and a few slices of ripe avocado on top. They're also good on top of a salad with a lemon-based vinaigrette or with a little Dijon mustard, honey mustard, or ketchup for dipping.

Sweet and Tangy Tuna Salad Lettuce Wraps

DAIRY-FREE, GLUTEN-FREE, NUT-FREE
SERVES: 4 | **PREP TIME:** 10 minutes

Tuna salad is a simple nutrient-dense option for a quick lunch or dinner. This version has some tangy apple and probiotic goodness for a flavor and nutrition boost. Tuna often contains mercury; limit your intake to once a week and choose brands that test to ensure the mercury levels are low, such as Safe Catch.

2 (5-ounce) cans no-salt-added tuna, packed in water, drained

¼ cup mayonnaise

½ Granny Smith apple, peeled and finely shredded

1 celery stalk, very finely diced

1 tablespoon sauerkraut, finely diced

2 teaspoons Dijon mustard

2 teaspoons minced garlic

Olive oil, for drizzling

Pinch ground black pepper

5 ounces romaine or butter leaf lettuce, whole leaves

1. In a medium bowl, mix together the tuna, mayonnaise, apple, celery, sauerkraut, mustard, garlic, a drizzle of olive oil, and a pinch of pepper until well combined. Taste and adjust the seasoning as desired.

2. For adults and older eaters, spoon 2 to 3 tablespoons of the tuna salad into one or two stacked lettuce leaves to use as a wrap.

3. Serve baby 2 to 4 tablespoons of the tuna salad on a plate or tray to eat with a fork or spoon. Store leftovers in an airtight container in the refrigerator for up to 5 days.

Mushroom and Leek Fried Eggs

GLUTEN-FREE, NUT-FREE, VEGETARIAN

MAKES: 4 eggs | **PREP TIME:** 10 minutes | **COOK TIME:** 15 minutes

Eggs are a great nutrient-dense and versatile protein. I love that they're a perfect vehicle for vegetables and can be enjoyed any time of the day. This version is quick and delicious for breakfast or a lighter dinner. We love them with a runny yolk, but if you prefer it more set, add a few minutes to the cook time.

3 tablespoons unsalted butter, cut into ½-inch chunks, divided

1 large leek, halved and very thinly sliced

4 ounces mushrooms, stems removed, halved, and thinly sliced

¼ teaspoon sea salt, divided

4 large eggs

Pinch ground black pepper

1. In a large skillet, melt 2 tablespoons of the butter over medium heat. Add the leek, mushrooms, and ⅛ teaspoon of the salt. Cook for about 5 minutes, or until the vegetables begin to brown and soften.

2. Spread the leeks and mushrooms out in an even layer and add the remaining chunks (1 tablespoon) of butter and allow to melt. Crack the eggs into the pan and season with the remaining ⅛ teaspoon salt and the pepper to taste. Cook for 3 to 4 minutes, or until the egg is set to your liking, then flip and cook for 1 minute more.

3. Let 1 egg and 2 tablespoons of vegetables cool, then give them to baby on a plate to eat with their hands or a fork. Store leftovers in an airtight container in the refrigerator for up to 4 days.

TIP: Try this with bell peppers or kale, and feel free to serve topped with fresh avocado slices and chopped cherry tomatoes.

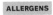

Butternut Squash Soup

DAIRY-FREE, GLUTEN-FREE

SERVES: 4+ | **PREP TIME:** 15 minutes | **COOK TIME:** 45 minutes

This soup was one of the first things I made after coming home from the hospital with our oldest. It was soothing and nourishing, didn't take a lot of effort, and was easy to freeze for leftovers. Then, my husband and I ate it out of coffee mugs. Now we eat it in bowls instead of mugs . . . mostly.

2 tablespoons coconut oil

1 medium sweet onion, chopped

1 small Granny Smith apple, peeled and chopped

1 celery stalk, chopped

1 large carrot, chopped

2 teaspoons minced garlic

2 teaspoons chopped fresh ginger

2 teaspoons turmeric

1 teaspoon ground cinnamon

4 cups 1-inch peeled butternut squash cubes, fresh or frozen

3 cups Slow Cooker Bone Broth (page 36) or store-bought bone broth

¼ cup cilantro leaves

1 can full-fat coconut milk

1. In a large stockpot, heat the oil over medium heat. Add the onion, apple, celery, and carrot and sauté for 5 to 8 minutes, or until soft. Add the garlic, ginger, turmeric, and cinnamon and cook for 1 minute more, or until fragrant.

2. Add the squash and broth, increase the heat to high, and bring the broth to a boil. Then turn down the heat to low and simmer for about 30 minutes, or until the squash is tender and can easily be pierced with a fork. Add the cilantro leaves.

3. If you have an immersion blender, puree until smooth. If not, carefully ladle the soup into your blender, in batches if necessary. Allow the steam to escape through the venting hole in the lid but cover it with a clean kitchen towel to avoid splatter. Blend until smooth.

4. Pour the blended soup back into the large pot. Stir in the coconut milk.

5. Let 2 to 4 tablespoons cool and serve to baby in a bowl to eat with a spoon. Store leftovers in an airtight container in the refrigerator for up to 4 days or in the freezer for up to 3 months.

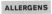ALLERGENS

Loaded Hummus

DAIRY-FREE, GLUTEN-FREE, NUT-FREE, VEGAN

SERVES: 4 | **PREP TIME:** 15 minutes

This is one of my family's favorite summer meals—no cooking, quick, and so good with fresh herbs and garden vegetables. Try adding caramelized onion, ground beef, and feta on top for a truly decadent meal.

1 batch Classic Hummus (page 42) or store-bought hummus (about 2 cups)

1 pint cherry tomatoes, quartered or thinly sliced

1 tablespoon thinly sliced fresh basil, mint, or a combination

¼ teaspoon sea salt

Pinch ground black pepper

Juice of ½ lemon

Olive oil, for drizzling

1 large cucumber, cut into ¼-inch rounds

1. Place the hummus in a large serving bowl or on a plate. Top with the cherry tomatoes, basil, salt, pepper, lemon juice, and a drizzle of olive oil.

2. Lay the cucumbers around the outside of the hummus to use as "chips" for scooping up the hummus. This is for adults and older children.

3. Serve baby 2 to 4 tablespoons of the Loaded Hummus (without the cucumbers) in a bowl to eat with a spoon. Store leftovers in an airtight container in the refrigerator for up to 4 days.

TIP: You may try cutting up the cucumber into matchsticks for baby to try, but their ability to chew them will depend on your child's skill level.

Powered-Up PB&J

DAIRY-FREE, VEGAN

MAKES: 1 sandwich | **PREP TIME:** 10 minutes

A good peanut butter and jelly sandwich is almost a childhood requirement. Even as an adult, I've had days where PB&J hits the spot. This is a powered-up version of the classic PB&J, so when your kid asks for it for the third (or millionth) time in a row, you actually feel good about saying yes.

2 pieces gluten-free or whole-grain bread

1 to 2 tablespoons Chia Seed Jam (page 68) or store-bought low-sugar jam sprinkled with 1 teaspoon chia seeds

1 to 2 tablespoons all-natural creamy peanut butter

1 teaspoon hemp seed

1 teaspoon ground flaxseed

1. On one slice of bread, spread the jam in an even layer.

2. On the other slice of the bread, spread an even layer of peanut butter and sprinkle with the hemp seed and ground flaxseed. Put the two halves together to close the sandwich.

3. Serve baby a quarter square of the sandwich or thin strips on a plate or tray to eat with their hands. Store leftovers in an airtight container in the refrigerator for up to 2 days.

TIP: For a peanut-free option, try all-natural creamy almond butter. Need a completely nut-free option? Try sunflower seed butter. For a jam-free option, use thinly cut banana slices sprinkled with chia seeds instead.

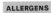

Delicata Squash Taco Boats

GLUTEN-FREE, NUT-FREE

SERVES: 4+ | **PREP TIME:** 10 minutes | **COOK TIME:** 45 minutes

These squash boats have the deliciousness of a taco with a lot more nutrients and no hard, choking-hazard shell. Feel free to eat or remove the peel of the squash. For your little one, base the removal of the peel on their eating skill level; if they're having trouble with the peel, you can always remove it during the meal, too.

2 large Delicata squash, ends trimmed, cut lengthwise, seeds and strings removed

2 tablespoons avocado oil

8 ounces ground beef

1 small sweet onion, peeled and finely diced

1 small bell pepper, any color, finely diced

1 teaspoon minced garlic

1 teaspoon paprika

½ teaspoon sea salt

½ teaspoon dried oregano

Pinch ground cinnamon

1 teaspoon ground cumin

1 (15-ounce) can no-salt-added black beans, rinsed and drained

½ cup salsa

1 cup shredded cheddar cheese

1 to 2 cups lettuce, shredded (optional)

¼ cup sour cream (optional)

½ ripe avocado, pitted and thinly sliced (optional)

1. Preheat the oven to 400°F. Line a baking sheet with parchment paper.

2. Lay the squash halves cut-side down on the prepared baking sheet and bake for 30 minutes, or until you can easily pierce the skin and flesh with a fork.

3. Meanwhile, in a large skillet, heat the oil over medium heat. Add the beef and cook for 3 to 5 minutes, stirring and breaking up the meat, until it begins to brown.

4. Add the onion and bell pepper and sauté for about 5 minutes, or until softened. Then stir in the garlic, paprika, salt, oregano, and cinnamon and cook for 1 minute more, or until fragrant. Stir in the beans and salsa, cooking for another 2 minutes, or until heated through.

5. When the squash halves are ready, carefully flip them over and evenly divide the beef mixture among the four halves. Evenly distribute the cheese over the four squash boats and bake for another 5 to 8 minutes, or until the cheese is melted and bubbly.

6. Let half of a squash boat cool, then cut it into bite-size pieces with the toppings on the side. Serve to baby on a plate or tray to eat with their hands or a fork. Store leftovers in an airtight container in the refrigerator for up to 4 days.

TIP: Use whatever fixings you would typically use for tacos. If you want a dairy-free version, skip the cheese. For a vegan option, use tofu or skip the meat all together. You can also use ground turkey or chicken.

Chicken Nuggets with a Boost

DAIRY-FREE, GLUTEN-FREE

SERVES: 4 | **PREP TIME:** 10 minutes | **COOK TIME:** 16 minutes

Another classic kid staple with a big nutrition boost—liver! Yes, you can omit the liver, but I highly recommend including it. It adds protein, iron, B vitamins, and more. These are made with a gluten-free coating that adds additional protein and healthy fats. I always wish I'd made a double batch; they are gone at our house quite quickly.

Avocado oil cooking spray

2 cups finely ground almond flour

1 pound ground chicken

1 to 2 ounces chicken liver, frozen and then grated, or 2 to 3 tablespoons Chicken Liver Pâté (page 52)

1 tablespoon finely minced chives

1 tablespoon dried parsley

Scant 1 teaspoon dried dill

1 teaspoon minced garlic

½ teaspoon sea salt

1. Preheat the oven to 400°F. Line a baking sheet with parchment paper and lightly spray the paper with avocado oil.

2. Put the almond flour in a small shallow bowl or pan.

3. In a large bowl, mix together the chicken, liver, chives, parsley, dill, garlic, and salt.

4. Scoop 1 to 2 tablespoons of the chicken mixture into your hands and form it into a nugget shape. Then dredge it in the almond flour and place it on the prepared baking sheet. Repeat this step with remaining chicken mixture, leaving about 1 inch between each nugget.

5. Lightly spray the tops of the chicken nuggets with cooking spray, then bake for 8 to 10 minutes, or until the underside is starting to brown. Flip the nuggets and bake for another 6 to 8 minutes, or until they are starting to turn golden and are cooked through.

6. Let one or two nuggets cool, cut them into strips or bite-size pieces, then serve to baby on a plate or tray to eat with their hands or a fork. Store leftovers in an airtight container in the refrigerator for up to 2 days.

TIP: Note that the liver may show up as "spots" in the cooked nuggets because it's a darker meat. If your little one is sensitive to how foods look and will be thrown by the "dots" in their nuggets, I recommend using the pâté instead of the grated liver.

Pesto Pasta

GLUTEN-FREE, NUT-FREE

SERVES: 4 | **PREP TIME:** 10 minutes | **COOK TIME:** 15 minutes

This dish was born out of desperation. We had some wilty greens that needed to be used, a bell pepper that had seen better days, and a leftover onion that was on its last leg. I needed dinner for ravenous, ready-to-mutiny kids, and this dish was born, quickly becoming almost a weekly staple.

2 tablespoons avocado oil

1 medium sweet onion, peeled, quartered, and very thinly sliced

Pinch sea salt

8 ounces chickpea pasta

1 cup peas, fresh or frozen

1 teaspoon minced garlic

1 small bell pepper, any color, finely diced

1 batch Simple Pesto (page 45) or store-bought pesto

½ cup shredded Parmesan cheese (optional)

1. Fill a large stockpot three-quarters full with water. Bring the water to a boil over high heat.

2. Meanwhile, in a medium skillet, heat the oil over medium heat. Add the onion and salt and sauté, stirring occasionally, for about 8 minutes, or until the onion begins to caramelize.

3. Once the water in the stockpot is boiling, add the pasta and cook according to the package instructions until al dente (8 to 10 minutes).

4. If the peas are frozen, add them to the pasta after it has cooked for about 5 minutes. (If fresh, skip this step.)

5. Once the onions are ready, add the garlic to the skillet and cook for 1 minute more, or until fragrant. Remove from the heat and set aside.

6. When pasta is cooked, drain it, then return it to the pot. Mix in the onions, bell pepper, and fresh peas, then the pesto. Stir gently to coat and evenly mix. Top with Parmesan, if using.

7. Let a ¼-cup portion cool, then chop everything up into bite-size pieces and serve to baby on a plate or tray to eat with their hands, a spoon, or a fork. Store leftovers in an airtight container in the refrigerator for up to 4 days.

TIP: This dish is incredibly versatile. Do you have mushrooms that need to be used? Sauté them with the onions. Have a bit of kale and some Swiss chard hanging out in your refrigerator? Use it for the pesto. Leftover sausage, pepperoni, chicken, or salami can also be chopped up and tossed in before serving.

Kale and Sausage Pizza Beans

GLUTEN-FREE, NUT-FREE

SERVES: 4+ | **PREP TIME:** 10 minutes | **COOK TIME:** 30 minutes

This vegetable-filled twist on pizza is an awesome way to get some of those greens that are a little harder for baby to chew into their diet. This is an easy one-pot meal if you have a large oven-safe skillet or cast-iron pan. Otherwise, transfer to an 8-by-8-inch baking dish before adding the cheese and baking.

2 tablespoons avocado oil

1 large sweet onion, diced

2 celery stalks, diced

1 large carrot, finely diced

4 ounces mushrooms, diced

3 to 4 ounces Italian sausage

¼ teaspoon sea salt

Pinch ground black pepper

2 teaspoons minced garlic

1 small bunch kale, thick stems removed and leaves finely chopped

1 tablespoon dried parsley

½ teaspoon dried basil

½ teaspoon dried oregano

1 (15-ounce) can tomato puree

2 (15-ounce) cans no-salt-added cannellini beans, rinsed and drained

½ cup Slow Cooker Bone Broth (page 36), store-bought broth, or water (optional)

2 cups shredded mozzarella cheese

½ cup shredded Parmesan cheese

1. Preheat the oven to 450°F.

2. In a large oven-safe skillet, heat the oil over medium-high heat. Add the onion, celery, carrot, mushrooms, and sausage, then season with salt and pepper. Cook for 8 to 10 minutes, stirring and breaking up the sausage, until lightly browned.

3. Add the garlic and cook for 1 minute, or until fragrant. Then add the kale, parsley, basil, and oregano and cook for another 2 minutes, or until the kale is starting to wilt.

4. Pour in the tomato puree and bring it to a simmer, then stir in the beans. If the mix looks dry, add broth ¼ cup at a time. Simmer for 10 minutes or until the sauce is just starting to thicken.

5. Sprinkle the cheeses over the top and transfer to the oven to cook for 10 to 15 minutes, or until the cheese is bubbly and starting to turn golden.

6. Let 2 to 4 tablespoons cool, then serve to baby on a plate or tray to eat with their hands or a spoon. Store leftovers in an airtight container in the refrigerator for up to 4 days.

TIP: This can also be made through step 4, cooled, transferred to an airtight container, and frozen for up to 3 months. Cook from frozen, foil-covered for about 45 minutes, then uncovered until heated through and bubbly, about 30 minutes more. Add the cheese in the last 10 to 15 minutes.

Kale and Sausage Crustless Quiche

GLUTEN-FREE, NUT-FREE
SERVES: 4+ | **PREP TIME:** 15 minutes | **COOK TIME:** 1 hour

A simple breakfast or dinner option rich in protein and choline, this dish creates an easy way to include leafy greens in your little one's diet. I love finding ways to incorporate greens like kale in recipes that make the bitterness less prominent.

2 teaspoons avocado oil, plus more for greasing

1 small sweet onion, peeled, halved, and thinly sliced

2 to 4 ounces mild Italian sausage (casings removed)

2 cups loosely packed kale, large stems removed and finely chopped

2 cups shredded fontina cheese

¾ cup full-fat plain unsweetened yogurt

5 large eggs

Pinch sea salt

Pinch ground black pepper

1. Preheat the oven to 375°F. Lightly grease an 8-by-8-inch or 9-inch cake pan.

2. In a large skillet, heat the oil over medium-low heat. Add the onion and cook, stirring occasionally, for 10 to 15 minutes, or until starting to caramelize.

3. Add the sausage to the pan, stirring and breaking up the meat, for about 5 minutes, or until the sausage starts to brown. Add the kale and cook for 2 to 3 minutes more, or until the kale starts to wilt.

4. Pour the sausage and vegetables into the prepared baking pan, spreading them evenly across the bottom, and sprinkle the cheese over the top.

5. In a large bowl, whisk together the yogurt, eggs, salt, and pepper. Pour the mixture over the top of the cheese, sausage, and vegetables.

6. Bake for 30 to 40 minutes, or until the quiche puffs up and is starting to brown and the eggs are completely set. Let cool for at least 5 minutes before serving.

7. Serve baby a 2-by-1-inch piece of quiche on a plate or tray to eat with their hands or a fork. Store leftovers in an airtight container in the refrigerator for up to 4 days.

TIP: This reheats beautifully. You can even make it ahead of time, cool completely to store in the refrigerator, and then reheat for 10 to 15 minutes in a 350°F oven. You can also heat individual portions for 1 to 2 minutes in the microwave. (Cook time will vary based on microwave strength.) Omit the sausage for a vegetarian option.

Curry Stuffed Peppers

DAIRY-FREE, GLUTEN-FREE, NUT-FREE

SERVES: 4 | **PREP TIME:** 15 minutes | **COOK TIME:** 45 minutes

Stuffed peppers are easy and adaptable. If you don't have all the vegetables listed, use the ones you do. If you have extra filling, you can cook it in a small ramekin to eat plain or with an egg over the top. If the pepper seems to be too challenging of a texture for your little one, simply serve them 2 to 4 tablespoons of the filling and omit the pepper entirely, or cut it into long strips for them to explore.

2 tablespoons avocado oil

1 medium sweet onion, finely diced

2 celery stalks, finely diced

4 ounces mushrooms, stems removed and diced

1 pound ground beef

3 ounces chicken liver, diced (optional)

1 tablespoon curry powder

1 teaspoon sea salt

½ teaspoon ground ginger

2 cups finely chopped spinach

1 cup Basic Cauliflower Rice (page 97) or store-bought riced cauliflower

3 large bell peppers, any color, halved and seeded

1. Preheat the oven to 400°F. Line a large baking sheet with parchment paper.

2. In a large skillet, heat the oil over medium heat. Add the onion, celery, and mushrooms and cook for 5 to 8 minutes, or until they begin to soften.

3. Add the beef, liver (if using), curry powder, salt, and ginger. Cook for 5 minutes, stirring and breaking up the meat, until the meat is browned.

4. Add the spinach and cauliflower rice, cooking and stirring for another 2 minutes, or until the spinach just begins to wilt. Remove from the heat.

5. Arrange the pepper halves on the prepared baking sheet, cut-side up. Fill them to the top with the filling, packing it down into the pepper with the back of the wooden spoon.

6. Bake for 20 to 30 minutes, or until the pepper begins to soften.

7. Cut one of the stuffed pepper halves in half, then cut into bite-size pieces, and let them cool. Serve to baby on a plate or in a bowl to eat with their hands or a fork. Store leftovers in an airtight container in the refrigerator for up to 3 days.

Sweet Potato Shepherd's Pie

DAIRY-FREE, GLUTEN-FREE, NUT-FREE
SERVES: 4+ | **PREP TIME:** 20 minutes | **COOK TIME:** 30 minutes

Shepherd's pie is an amazing comfort food but typically not so nutritious. This version has become a staple in my house for cold evenings. Bake the sweet potatoes at 400°F, wrapped in foil, until pierced easily with a fork, 45 to 60 minutes. Alternatively, pierce the sweet potatoes three or four times with a fork and microwave for 5 to 8 minutes on high until soft. Allow them to cool while preparing the filling.

4 tablespoons avocado oil, divided

1 large sweet onion, diced

3 or 4 carrots, diced

8 ounces mushrooms, stems removed and diced

1 cup peas, fresh or frozen

2 teaspoons minced garlic

1 pound ground beef

3 ounces chicken liver, finely chopped (optional)

3 to 4 cups finely chopped fresh spinach, or 1 cup frozen chopped spinach

½ to 1 cup Slow Cooker Bone Broth (page 36), store-bought broth, or water

1 tablespoon ketchup or tomato paste with a splash apple cider vinegar

1 teaspoon gluten-free tamari

2 teaspoons ground flaxseed

1 to 2 teaspoons dried rosemary, finely chopped

1 to 2 teaspoons dried thyme

½ teaspoon ground black pepper, divided

Pinch sea salt

2 large sweet potatoes, cooked and cooled

1 large egg

1. Preheat the oven to 400°F. Line an 8-by-8-inch baking dish with parchment paper.

2. In a large skillet, heat 2 tablespoons of oil over medium-high heat. Add the onion and carrots and sauté for about 5 minutes, or until they begin to soften. Add the mushrooms, peas, garlic, ground beef, and liver. Cook for 5 to 7 minutes, stirring and breaking up the meat, until the meat is browned and cooked through.

3. Add the spinach, broth, ketchup, tamari, flaxseed, rosemary, thyme, ¼ teaspoon of pepper, and the salt. Increase the heat to high and bring to a boil. Then turn down the heat to low and simmer for 10 minutes, or until the filling has thickened slightly. Spread the filling into the prepared baking dish.

4. Scoop the sweet potato flesh into a medium bowl. Add the egg, the remaining 2 tablespoons of oil, and the remaining ¼ teaspoon of pepper, and season with salt. Mash and mix until mostly smooth, then spread the mixture on top of the filling in an even layer.

5. Bake for 40 to 45 minutes, or until heated through. Let the shepherd's pie cool for 5 minutes before serving.

6. Serve baby 2 to 4 tablespoons on their plate or in a bowl to eat with a spoon. Store leftovers in an airtight container in the refrigerator for up to 5 days.

TIP: To make ahead, after step 4, cover with parchment paper, then foil, and freeze for up to 3 months. To reheat, bake at 400°F for 1 hour, covered, then 20 to 30 minutes, uncovered, until completely heated through.

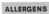

Greek-Inspired Lamb Cauliflower Rice Bowls

GLUTEN-FREE, NUT-FREE

SERVES: 4 to 6 | **PREP TIME:** 20 minutes | **COOK TIME:** 15 minutes

One of my family's favorite weeknight dinners comes together in a flash if you have a batch of Lamb Oven Meatballs in the freezer and leftover Classic Hummus, and Basic Cauliflower Rice on hand. If not, whip the meatballs up quickly and pop them in the oven before prepping the rest of the ingredients. Use store-bought hummus and riced cauliflower, cooked according to the package directions, to speed things up.

1 batch Basic Cauliflower Rice (page 97) or store-bought riced cauliflower

½ to 1 small cucumber, cut paper-thin

2 cups cherry tomatoes, quartered

4 ounces goat cheese

1 batch Classic Hummus (page 42) or store-bought hummus

Fresh mint or basil (optional)

1 batch Lamb Oven Meatballs (page 141)

1. In a large pan, cook the cauliflower rice for about 5 minutes, or to your desired tenderness.

2. Portion the cauliflower rice into bowls or onto plates. For adults and older eaters, top with cucumber, cherry tomatoes, a quarter of the goat cheese, 1 to 2 tablespoons of hummus, and a sprinkling of fresh herbs (if using). Add the cooked meatballs and serve.

3. For baby, serve the dish deconstructed: Cut one or two meatballs into quarters and serve alongside 1 or 2 tablespoons of cauliflower rice, 1 tablespoon of hummus, tomatoes, and goat cheese, broken up into bite-size pieces to be eaten with their hands or a spoon. Store leftovers separately to prevent things from getting soggy. Meatballs and rice can be stored together, and everything will keep in the refrigerator for up to 4 days.

TIP: The thinly sliced cucumbers are better for kiddos who are at least a year old. It depends on your child's unique feeding skills.

Homemade Burrito Bowls

GLUTEN-FREE, NUT-FREE
SERVES: 4 | **PREP TIME:** 15 minutes | **COOK TIME:** 15 minutes

We eat a lot of "bowls" in my family. I find them to be a great way to get in a well-balanced meal without having to make several different dishes to accomplish it. This bowl is inspired by the Chipotle Mexican Grill burrito bowls that my family loves. For the little ones, I recommend serving this kind of meal "deconstructed" so that each part of the dish that's appropriate for your little one's skill level is plated separately from another part. This allows your child to explore mixing (or *not*) the food on their own and exploring at their own pace.

For the burrito bowls

2 tablespoons avocado oil, divided

1 batch Basic Cauliflower Rice (page 97) or store-bought riced cauliflower

Zest of 1 lime

½ teaspoon sea salt, divided

¼ teaspoon ground black pepper, divided

1 small yellow onion, finely diced

1 large bell pepper, any color, chopped

1 heaping teaspoon minced garlic

1 pound ground beef

½ teaspoon dried oregano

½ teaspoon ground cumin

1 (15-ounce) can no-salt-added black or pinto beans, rinsed and drained

For the toppings

½ to 1 cup shredded cheese of choice (optional)

1 cup Simple Guacamole (page 41) or Kale Guacamole (page 69) (optional)

¼ cup sour cream (optional)

1 to 2 cups shredded lettuce (optional)

½ cup diced tomatoes (optional)

½ cup salsa (optional)

1 cup roasted corn (optional)

TO MAKE THE BURRITO BOWLS

1. In a large skillet, heat 1 tablespoon of the oil over medium heat. Add the cauli-flower rice, lime zest, ¼ teaspoon of salt, and ⅛ teaspoon black pepper. Cook for about 5 minutes, or to your desired tenderness. Transfer to a small bowl.

2. In the same skillet, heat the remaining 1 tablespoon of oil over medium-high heat. Add the onion and bell pepper and sauté for 3 to 5 minutes, or until they begin to soften. Stir in the garlic and cook for 1 minute more, or until fragrant.

3. Add the beef, oregano, and cumin and cook for 5 to 8 minutes, stirring and break-ing up the meat, until the meat is browned and cooked through. Mix in the beans and cook for 2 to 3 minutes, or until the beans are heated through.

TO TOP THE BOWLS

4. For adults and older eaters, start with a base of the rice, add the meat mixture, and then add any desired toppings. Serve baby 1 tablespoon of each on a plate to eat with their hands or a spoon. Store leftovers in an airtight container in the refrigerator for up to 4 days.

Cheeseburger Bowls

GLUTEN-FREE, NUT-FREE

SERVES: 4+ | **PREP TIME:** 15 minutes | **COOK TIME:** 20 minutes

This has become a nearly weekly staple in our house. My husband *loves* cheeseburgers, and I love feeding people things they love. I also love making sure our family is getting lots of vegetables and nutrient-rich foods. This was a compromise—one he hasn't complained about one bit.

For the burger bowls

2 tablespoons avocado oil, divided

1 medium sweet onion, halved and thinly sliced

6 to 8 ounces mushrooms, stems removed and chopped

½ teaspoon sea salt, divided

1 pound ground beef

½ teaspoon ground cumin

½ teaspoon paprika

Pinch ground black pepper

For the sauce

½ cup mayonnaise

1 heaping tablespoon ketchup

1 tablespoon mustard of choice

2 tablespoons dill sauerkraut, finely chopped

For the toppings

1 small head cabbage, shredded

1 cup cherry tomatoes, quartered or thinly sliced

½ cup shredded cheddar cheese

¼ cup dill sauerkraut

TO MAKE THE BURGER BOWLS

1. In a large skillet, heat 1 tablespoon of the oil over medium heat. Add the onion, mushrooms, and ¼ teaspoon of the salt and sauté for about 8 minutes, or until the vegetables have softened and browned. Transfer to a small bowl.

2. Pour the remaining 1 tablespoon of oil into the same skillet, then add the ground beef, cumin, paprika, remaining ¼ teaspoon salt, and the pepper. Cook for 5 minutes, stirring and breaking up the meat, until the meat is browned. Remove from the heat.

TO MAKE THE SAUCE

3. In a small bowl, whisk together the mayonnaise, ketchup, mustard, and sauerkraut.

TO TOP THE BOWLS

4. For adults and older eaters, place a good handful of cabbage into individual bowls, top with ground meat, then the onions and mushrooms, and finally tomatoes, cheese, and sauerkraut. Drizzle some sauce over the top of each serving. Serve baby about 1 tablespoon of each (except the cabbage) separately on a plate to eat with their hands or a fork. Store leftovers in separate airtight containers in the refrigerator for up to 3 days.

TIP: This is awesome with the Rosemary Garlic Sweet Potato Fries (page 48). You can also omit the cheese for a dairy-free option and change up the toppings for your own family's favorites.

Sweet Potato Pizza Skillet

GLUTEN-FREE, NUT-FREE

SERVES: 4 | **PREP TIME:** 10 minutes | **COOK TIME:** 35 minutes

This gluten-free, nutrient-rich pizza-inspired option is easier for little ones to eat, as pizza crust can be quite chewy and tricky. We love this with some of our classic topping favorites, such as black olives and pepperoni, but make it your own with whatever toppings you like best. You can opt to either shred the sweet potatoes, or if you have a spiralizer, that works beautifully, too. Make sure the pepperoni has no nitrates added.

2 tablespoons avocado oil

3 medium or 2 large sweet potatoes, grated

1 small yellow onion, finely diced

1 heaping teaspoon minced garlic

1 teaspoon dried basil

½ teaspoon dried oregano

Pinch sea salt

Pinch ground black pepper

1 (15-ounce) no-salt-added tomato sauce or puree

1 cup shredded mozzarella cheese

¼ cup Parmesan cheese

1 small bell pepper, any color, finely chopped

⅓ cup black olives, chopped or thinly sliced

4 ounces pepperoni, chopped

1. Preheat the oven to 425°F.

2. In a large oven-safe skillet or cast-iron pan, heat the oil over medium heat. Add the sweet potatoes and onion. Cook, stirring occasionally, for about 5 minutes, or until both begin to soften.

3. Add the garlic, basil, oregano, salt, and black pepper. Stir and cook for about 1 minute more, or until fragrant. Stir in the tomato sauce. Remove from the heat.

4. Sprinkle the mozzarella and Parmesan evenly over the sweet potato mix, then sprinkle the bell pepper, olives, and pepperoni over the cheeses.

5. Bake for 20 to 25 minutes, or until the cheese has melted and is starting to brown in spots.

6. Let 2 to 4 tablespoons cool, then serve to baby on a plate or in a bowl for them to eat with their hands or a spoon. Store leftovers in an airtight container in the refrigerator for up to 4 days.

Baking Sheet Chicken and Veggies

DAIRY-FREE, GLUTEN-FREE, NUT-FREE

SERVES: 4 | **PREP TIME:** 15 minutes | **COOK TIME:** 30 minutes

I love one-pan meals. It means less time over the stove and fewer dishes to wash. This one is a great, adaptable base recipe: add some barbeque sauce or pesto or even melt some cheese over the top of the chicken to change it up.

4 (4-ounce) boneless, skinless chicken breasts

½ teaspoon sea salt, divided

¼ teaspoon ground black pepper, divided

8 ounces baby red potatoes, quartered

8 ounces fresh green beans, ends trimmed and halved crosswise

2 tablespoons avocado oil

2 heaping teaspoons minced garlic

1 teaspoon dried basil

1 teaspoon dried thyme

1. Preheat the oven to 400°F. Line a large baking sheet with parchment paper.

2. Season the chicken breasts with ¼ teaspoon of salt and ⅛ teaspoon of pepper, then place them in a single layer on one side of the prepared baking sheet.

3. In a large bowl, combine the potatoes, green beans, oil, garlic, basil, and thyme and toss until the vegetables are evenly coated. Then spread the seasoned vegetables in a single layer on the other half of the pan.

4. Bake for 20 to 30 minutes, or until the chicken is cooked through and the potatoes are golden and easily pierced with a fork.

5. Let cool 2 tablespoons of chicken, cut into bite-size chunks or strips, a few pieces of potato, and a green bean or two. Serve to baby on a plate or tray to eat with their hands or a fork. Store leftovers in an airtight container in the refrigerator for up to 4 days.

TIP: Try topping the chicken with mozzarella and Parmesan for the last few minutes and serving with the Tomato Basil Salad (page 124). You could also use store-bought pesto or the Simple Pesto (page 45) for a quick, easy sauce.

Open-Faced Grilled Cheese with a Twist

NUT-FREE, VEGETARIAN

MAKES: 1 slice | **PREP TIME:** 10 minutes | **COOK TIME:** 10 minutes

One of my goals when working with kids and families is to take the classic dishes of childhood and make them more nutritious. Treats and food just for fun, not nutrition, are absolutely okay every once in a while, but I think if we can find ways to have some of the favorites without sacrificing nutrition, then why not?

1 tablespoon unsalted butter, softened

1 slice gluten-free or whole-grain bread

1 to 2 tablespoons Kale Guacamole (page 69)

½ cup shredded cheddar cheese

1. Turn the broiler on to high. Heat a medium oven-safe skillet over medium heat.

2. Spread an even layer of butter on one side of the bread. On the other side, spread a layer of the guacamole. Lay the bread butter-side down in the hot pan. Sprinkle the cheese evenly over the guacamole.

3. Cook for 2 to 4 minutes, or until the bottom of the bread is just starting to turn golden. Transfer the pan to the oven under the broiler and broil for 1 to 2 minutes, or until the cheese has melted and is bubbly.

4. Let a quarter square of the cheesy bread cool. If needed, cut it into thin strips, then serve to baby on a plate or tray to eat with their hands. Store leftovers in an airtight container in the refrigerator for up to 2 days.

TIP: This is a real winner alongside the Butternut Squash Soup (page 162). With older eaters, feel free to skip the broiler and make a full grilled cheese sandwich on the stove; I find for most new eaters, the thickness of a full grilled cheese is too much for them to safely or comfortably chew.

Beef and Sweet Potato Tacos

GLUTEN-FREE, NUT-FREE

SERVES: 4 | **PREP TIME:** 15 minutes | **COOK TIME:** 25 minutes

Taco night is beloved at my house. We make different taco variations, but this is a steadfast favorite from way back in our pre-kid days. It's been fun to introduce our little ones to it; plus, everything but the cabbage is a great texture for baby.

1 large sweet potato, cut into ½-inch chunks

2 tablespoons avocado oil, divided

1 teaspoon ground cumin, divided

½ teaspoon paprika

½ teaspoon sea salt, divided

Pinch cayenne (optional)

12 corn tortillas

1 pound ground beef

1 small sweet onion, finely diced

Pinch ground black pepper

2 cups shredded cabbage

¼ cup fresh cilantro leaves

Juice of 1 lime

¼ cup diced Peppadew peppers, for topping (optional)

1 ripe avocado, chopped into ½-inch chunks, for topping (optional)

4 tablespoons goat cheese, for topping (optional)

1. Preheat the oven to 400°F. Line a large baking sheet with parchment paper.

2. In a medium bowl, mix together the sweet potato, 1 tablespoon of the oil, ½ teaspoon of the cumin, the paprika, ¼ teaspoon of salt, and cayenne (if using). Toss gently to combine, then spread evenly on the prepared baking sheet.

3. Bake for 20 to 25 minutes, or until tender and starting to brown. In the last 2 minutes of cooking, add the tortillas to the oven to warm slightly before serving.

4. Meanwhile, in a large skillet, heat the remaining 1 tablespoon of oil over medium heat. Add the beef, onion, remaining ½ teaspoon of cumin, the remaining ¼ teaspoon of salt, and the black pepper. Sauté for about 8 minutes, or until the beef has browned and the onions are slightly soft. Remove from the heat.

5. In a medium bowl, mix together the cabbage, cilantro, and lime juice. Toss to combine.

6. For adults and older eaters, load the tortillas with the beef, sweet potatoes, cabbage mixture, and any of the desired toppings. Serve baby a few chunks of sweet potato, avocado, and goat cheese with a heaping tablespoon of the meat and a strip or two of the tortilla, all separately on a plate or tray to eat with their hands or a fork. Store leftovers in separate airtight containers in the refrigerator for up to 3 days.

TIP: Feel free to offer your little one a Peppadew pepper—they're sweet with a bit of spice, which some young eaters may enjoy.

Measurement Conversions

VOLUME EQUIVALENTS	U.S. STANDARD	U.S. STANDARD (OUNCES)	METRIC (APPROXIMATE)
LIQUID	2 tablespoons	1 fl. oz.	30 mL
	¼ cup	2 fl. oz.	60 mL
	½ cup	4 fl. oz.	120 mL
	1 cup	8 fl. oz.	240 mL
	1½ cups	12 fl. oz.	355 mL
	2 cups or 1 pint	16 fl. oz.	475 mL
	4 cups or 1 quart	32 fl. oz.	1 L
	1 gallon	128 fl. oz.	4 L
DRY	⅛ teaspoon	–	0.5 mL
	¼ teaspoon	–	1 mL
	½ teaspoon	–	2 mL
	¾ teaspoon	–	4 mL
	1 teaspoon	–	5 mL
	1 tablespoon	–	15 mL
	¼ cup	–	59 mL
	⅓ cup	–	79 mL
	½ cup	–	118 mL
	⅔ cup	–	156 mL
	¾ cup	–	177 mL
	1 cup	–	235 mL
	2 cups or 1 pint	–	475 mL
	3 cups	–	700 mL
	4 cups or 1 quart	–	1 L
	½ gallon	–	2 L
	1 gallon	–	4 L

OVEN TEMPERATURES

FAHRENHEIT	CELSIUS (APPROXIMATE)
250°F	120°C
300°F	150°C
325°F	165°C
350°F	180°C
375°F	190°C
400°F	200°C
425°F	220°C
450°F	230°C

WEIGHT EQUIVALENTS

U.S. STANDARD	METRIC (APPROXIMATE)
½ ounce	15 g
1 ounce	30 g
2 ounces	60 g
4 ounces	115 g
8 ounces	225 g
12 ounces	340 g
16 ounces or 1 pound	455 g

Resources

EATING SUPPLIES

Bumkins Splat Mat (Amazon.com)

Clean Cub Baby Led Weaning Long Sleeve Apron Bib (Amazon.com)

EZTOTZ baby utensils (Amazon.com)

Happy Kid and Happy Tot Superfood Protein and Fiber Bars and Superfood Pouches (Amazon.com; Target.com)

Munchkin Click Lock Weighted Straw Cup (Amazon.com; Target.com)

Squeasy Snacker Pouch (Amazon.com)

ONLINE RETAILERS FOR ORGANIC PRODUCTS

Butcher Box (ButcherBox.com)

Misfits Market (MisfitsMarket.com)

Thrive Market (ThriveMarket.com)

WEBSITES FOR RECIPES AND SUPPORT

The Ellen Satter Institute: "Raise a Healthy Child Who Is a Joy to Feed" (EllynSatterInstitute.org/how-to-feed/the-division-of-responsibility-in-feeding)

Environmental Working Group: "EWG's 2021 Shopper's Guide to Pesticides in Produce" (EWG.org/foodnews/summary.php)

Growing Independent Eaters (GIEaters.com)

Kids Eat in Color (KidsEatInColor.com)

Lily Nichols, RDN, CDE: "The Suprisingly Weak Evidence for Infant Sodium Requirements" (LilyNicholsRDN.com/salt-baby-food-infant-sodium-requirements)

References

Bakke, A. J., et al. "Mary Poppins Was Right: Adding Small Amounts of Sugar or Salt Reduces the Bitterness of Vegetables." *Appetite* 126 (July 2018): 90–101.

Barański, M., et al. "Higher Antioxidant and Lower Cadmium Concentrations and Lower Incidence of Pesticide Residues in Organically Grown Crops: A Systematic Literature Review and Meta-Analyses." *British Journal of Nutrition* 112, no. 5 (September 2014): 794–811.

Bouohlal, S., et al. "'Just a Pinch of Salt.' an Experimental Comparison of the Effect of Repeated Exposure and Flavor—Flavor Learning with Salt or Spice on Vegetable Acceptance in Toddlers." *Appetite* 83 (December 2014): 209–17.

Brown, A., and M. Lee. "A Descriptive Study Investigating the Use and Nature of Baby-Led Weaning In a UK Sample of Mothers." *Maternal and Child Nutrition* 7, no. 1 (January 2011): 34–47.

Brown, A., et al. "Baby-Led Weaning: The Evidence to Date." *Current Nutrition Reports* 6, no. 2 (2017): 148–56.

Cameron, S. L., et al. "Development and Pilot Testing Of Baby-Led Introduction to Solids—a Version of Baby-Led Weaning Modified to Address Concerns about Iron Deficiency, Growth Faltering and Choking." *BMC Pediatrics* 15, no. 9 (August 2015): DOI: 10.1186/s12887-015-0422-8.

Cameron, S. L., et al. "How Feasible Is Baby-Led Weaning as an Approach to Infant Feeding? A Review of the Evidence." *Nutrients* 4, no. 11 (November 2012): 1575–609.

Carruth, B. R., et al. "Prevalence of Picky Eaters among Infants and Toddlers and Their Caregivers' Decisions about Offering a New Food." *Journal of American Dietetic Association* 104, no. 1 Suppl 1 (January 2004): s57–s64.

Caton, S. J., et al. "Learning to Eat Vegetables in Early Life: The Role of Timing, Age and Individual Eating Traits." *PLoS ONE* 9, no. 5 (May 2014): e97609.

Chiu, Y. H., et al. "Association Between Pesticide Residue Intake from Consumption of Fruits and Vegetables and Pregnancy Outcomes Among Women Undergoing Infertility Treatment With Assisted Reproductive Technology." *JAMA Internal Medicine* 178, no 1 (January 2018): 17–26.

Clark, K. M., et al. "Breastfeeding, Mixed, or Formula Feeding at 9 Months of Age and the Prevalence of Iron Deficiency and Iron Deficiency Anemia in Two Cohorts of Infants in China." *Journal of Pediatrics* 181 (February 2017): 56–61.

Cuhra, M. "Review Of GMO Safety Assessment Studies: Glyphosate Residues in Roundup Ready Crops Is an Ignored Issue." *Environmental Sciences Europe* 27, no. 20 (September 2015): DOI.org/10.1186/s12302-015-0052-7.

Čukuranović, R., and S. Vlajković. "Age Related Anatomical and Functional Characteristics of Human Kidney." *Medicine and Biology* 12, no. 2 (2005): 61–69.

D'Auria, E., et al. "Baby-Led Weaning: What a Systematic Review Of the Literature Adds On." *Italian Journal of Pediatrics* 44, no. 1 (May 2018): 49.

DiNicolantonio, J. J., and S. C. Lucan. "The Wrong White Crystals: Not Salt but Sugar as Aetiological in Hypertension and Cardiometabolic Disease." *Open Heart* 1 (2014): e000167.

Emmerik, N. E., et al. "Dietary Intake of Sodium during Infancy and the Cardiovascular Consequences Later in Life: A Scoping Review." *Annals of Nutrition and Metabolism* 76, no. 2 (June 2020): 114–21.

Farina, W. M., et al. "Effects of the Herbicide Glyphosate on Honey Bee Sensory and Cognitive Abilities: Individual Impairments with Implications for the Hive." *Insects* 10, no. 10 (October 2019): 354.

Fewtrell, M., et al. "Complementary Feeding: A Position Paper by the European Society of Paediatric Gastroenterology, Hepatology, and Nutrition (ESPGHAN) Committee on Nutrition." *Journal of Pediatric Gastroenterology and Nutrition* 64, no. 1 (January 2017): 119–32.

Gill, J. P., et al. "Glyphosate Toxicity for Animals." *Environmental Chemistry Letters* 16, no. 2 (December 2017): 401–26.

Goldbohm, R. A., et al. "Food Consumption and Nutrient Intake by Children Aged 10 to 48 Months Attending Day Care in the Netherlands." *Nutrients* 8.7 (2016): 428.

Griffin, I. J., and S. A. Abrams. "Iron and Breastfeeding." *Pediatric Clinic of North America* 48, no. 2 (April 2001): 401–13.

Ha, S. K. "Dietary Salt Intake and Hypertension." *Electrolytes & Blood Pressure* 12, no. 1 (June 2014): 7–18.

Halpern, M. D., and P. W. Denning. "The Role of Intestinal Epithelial Barrier Function in the Development of NEC." *Tissue Barriers* 3, no. 1–2 (2015): e1000707.

Hessler, Uwe. "What's Driving Europe's Stance on Glyphosate." DW Academie (June 25, 2020). DW.com/en/whats-driving-europes-stance-on-glyphosate/a-53924882.

Hong, J., et al. "Breastfeeding and Red Meat Intake Are Associated with Iron Status in Healthy Korean Weaning-Age Infants." *Journal of Korean Medical Science* 32, no. 6 (June 2017): 974–84.

Karsten, H. D., et al. "Vitamins A, E and Fatty Acid Composition of the Eggs of Caged Hens and Pastured Hens." *Cambridge University Press* 25, no. 1 (March 2010): 45–54.

Koifman, S., et al. "Human Reproductive System Disturbances and Pesticide Exposure in Brazil." *Cadernos de Saúde Pública* 18, no. 2 (2002): 435–45.

Krebs, N. F. "Meat as an Early Complementary Food for Infants: Implications for Macro- And Micronutrient Intakes." *Nestle Nutrition Institute Workshop Series: Pediatric Program* 60 (2007): 221–33.

Krebs, N. F., and J. Westcott. "Zinc and Breastfed Infants: If and When Is There a Risk of Deficiency?" *Advances in Experimental Medicine and Biology* 503 (2002): 69–75.

Kuhn, J., et al. "Free-Range Farming: A Natural Alternative to Produce Vitamin D-Enriched Eggs." *Nutrition* 30, no. 4 (April 2014): 481–84.

Kuo, A. A., et al. "Introduction of Solid Food to Young Infants." *Maternal and Child Health Journal* 15, no. 8 (November 2011): 1185–194.

Lam, J. "Picky Eating in Children." *Frontiers in Pediatrics* 3, no. 41 (2015): DOI: 10.3389/fped.2015.00041.

Maier-Noth, A., et al. "The Lasting Influences of Early Food-Related Variety Experience: A Longitudinal Study of Vegetable Acceptance from 5 Months to 6 Years in Two Populations." *PLoS ONE* 11, no. 3 (March 2016): e0151356.

Malik, A. H., et al. "Impact of Sugar-Sweetened Beverages on Blood Pressure." *American Journal of Cardiology* 113, no. 9 (May 2014): 1574–80.

Motta, E. V. S., et al. "Glyphosate Perturbs the Gut Microbiota of Honey Bees." *PNAS* 115, no. 41 (October 2018): 10305–10.

Naylor, A. J., and A. L. Morrow. "Developmental Readiness of Normal Full Term Infants to Progress from Exclusive Breastfeeding to the Introduction of Complementary Foods." Linkages, Academy for Educational Development and the United States Agency for International Development (April 2001): pdf.usaid.gov/pdf_docs/Pnacs461.pdf.

Nicolopoulou-Stamati, P., et al. "Chemical Pesticides and Human Health: The Urgent Need for a New Concept in Agriculture." *Frontiers in Public Health* 4 (2016): 148.

Parigi, S. M., et al. "Breastmilk and Solid Food Shaping Intestinal Immunity." *Frontiers in Immunology* 19 (August 201): DOI.org/10.3389/fimmu.2015.00415.

Pase, M. P., et al. "Habitual Intake of Fruit Juice Predicts Central Blood Pressure." *Appetite* 84 (January 2015): 68–72.

Payau, F. A., and L. P. Hampton. "Salt Content of the Modern Diet." *The American Journal of Diseases of Children* 111, no.4 (1966): 370–373.

Prell, C., and B. Koletzko. "Breastfeeding and Complementary Feeding." *Deutsches Arzteblatt International* 113, no. 25 (June 2016): 435-44.

Rowan, H., and C. Harris. "Baby-LED Weaning and the Family Diet. A Pilot Study." *Appetite* 58, no. 3 (June 2012): 1046-49.

Samsel, A., and S. Seneff. "Glyphosate's Suppression of Cytochrome P450 Enzymes and Amino Acid Biosynthesis by the Gut Microbiome: Pathways to Modern Diseases." *Entropy* 15, no. 4 (April 2013): 1416-63.

Satter, Ellyn. "Ellyn Satter's Division of Responsibility in Feeding." The Ellen Satter Institute. EllynSatterInstitute.org/wp-content/uploads/2016/11/handout-dor-tasks-cap-2016.pdf.

Sevenhuysen, G. P., et al. "Developmental of Salivary a-Amylase in Infants from Birth to 5 Months." *American Journal of Clinical Nutrition* 39, no. 4 (1984): 584–88.

Stein, L. J., et al. "The Development of Salty Taste Acceptance Is Related to Dietary Experience in Human Infants: A Prospective Study." *American Journal of Clinical Nutrition* 95, no. 1 (January 2012): 123–29.

Whitten, C. F., and R.A. Stewart. "The Effect of Dietary Sodium in Infancy on Blood Pressure and Related Factors: Studies of Infants Fed Salted and Unsalted Diets for Five Months at Eight Months and Eight Years of Age." *Acta Pædiatrica* 69 (1980): 3–17.

Wright, C. M., et al. "Is Baby-Led Weaning Feasible? When Do Babies First Reach Out for and Eat Finger Foods?" *Maternal and Child Nutrition* 7, no. 1 (January 2011): 27–33.

Xi, B., et al. "Sugar-Sweetened Beverages and Risk of Hypertension and Cvd: A Dose-Response Meta-Analysis." *British Journal of Nutrition* 113, no. 5 (March 2015): 709–17.

Index

Acknowledgments

This book couldn't have happened without the encouragement and support of my amazing husband. Thank you for trying oh so many experimental recipes for the last decade. Thank you for being an amazing father to our children and willingly taking over childcare duties on weekends and evenings to enable me to pursue my own professional ambitions while still being the momma I want to be. You have held space for me and my dreams even when I haven't been sure how to fill that space. To my mother, thank you for spending retirement corralling my crazies so I can get a few hours of uninterrupted work done. And thank you to both my parents for fostering in me a desire to teach others and share my light, and for my love of food. You made family meals a priority and expectation and showed me from the beginning the power of good food, good conversation, and the family table.

About the Author

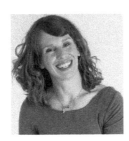 **Aubrey Phelps, MS, RDN, CLC,** is a registered functional dietitian/nutritionist, perinatal fitness coach, lactation counselor, kangaroula, and advocate for women as they make the journey into motherhood. Specializing in perinatal and pediatric nutrition, Aubrey supports clients working to grow their family from conception and a healthy pregnancy, through postpartum and infant feeding. She helps families get their little one off to the right start with nutrition and health, and those struggling with the anxiety of a child who isn't growing as expected. Aubrey believes motherhood is hard enough; feeding your little one shouldn't be! Her own personal and professional experiences with traumatic births, miscarriages, feeding issues and feeding tubes, premature birth, C-sections, and VBA2C have made Aubrey an expert in nourishing little ones from before birth to adolescence and beyond. She works as a consulting dietitian for Growing Independent Eaters, a home-based tube-weaning program, and is the owner of Matrescence Nutrition. To learn more, visit MatrescenceNutrition.com.